Articulation and Phonological Disorders

Articulation and Phonological Disorders

Assessment and Treatment Resource Manual

Adriana Peña-Brooks

M. N. Hegde

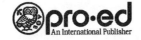
pro·ed
An International Publisher

8700 Shoal Creek Boulevard
Austin, Texas 78757-6897
800/897-3020 Fax: 800/397-7633
www.proedinc.com

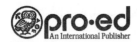

© 2007 by PRO-ED, Inc.
8700 Shoal Creek Boulevard
Austin, Texas 78757-6897
800/897-3202   Fax 800/397-7633
www.proedinc.com

Art Director: Jason Crosier
Designer: Kim Worley
This book is designed in Fairfield LH and Frutiger.

Printed in the United States of America

1   2   3   4   5   6   7   8   9   10   10   09   08   07   06

I dedicate this book to God for giving me the endurance to accomplish things that I believe impossible. To my husband, Ryan Brooks, who supports me in everything I do. To my beautiful two-year-old triplets, Jordan, Jacob, and Nolan, who, although not very cooperative and patient during preparation of this project, have been my daily inspiration. And to my mother, Maria Peña, who from an early age taught me the importance of strength and character.

—APB

Contents

◆　◆　◆　◆　◆　◆　◆　◆　◆　◆　◆　◆　◆

Introduction to the Manual and the Accompanying CD

◆   ◆   ◆   ◆   ◆   ◆   ◆   ◆   ◆   ◆   ◆   ◆   ◆

Articulation and Phonological Disorders: Assessment and Treatment Resource Manual was designed for practicing clinicians and students in communicative sciences and disorders working with children with articulation and phonological delays. The clinical materials in the *Manual* are most appropriate for school-age children from kindergarten to eighth grade, and because the school-based clinician services the majority of children with articulation and phonological disorders, they were tailored to that setting but are still appropriate for all clinical settings.

This *Manual* accompanies our textbook, *Assessment and Treatment of Articulation and Phonological Disorders in Children—Second Edition*. Therefore, the *Manual* does not contain the kinds of information that are typically included in a textbook. The *Manual* also omits articulation picture cards, word game boards, craft worksheets, and so forth that are readily available in countless commercial resources. The *Manual* offers a variety of clinical management materials such as data recording sheets, screening forms, sound establishment techniques, sound word exemplar lists, sample reports, parent and teacher letters, and so forth in one convenient source. Our goal was to develop a compilation of modifiable and printable assessment and treatment materials that could help simplify the clinician's professional life.

Each practical material is preceded by a quick introduction, which the clinician may skip if desired as they were written to stand independent of their introduction. With that said, the information could prove helpful, and we recommend that it be reviewed as necessary. Also, if the clinician needs more information on a particular topic addressed in the introductory sections, he or she may refer to the *Manual*'s accompanying textbook. We make frequent references to the textbook chapters in which additional information can be found. To simplify our writing, we refer to the textbook as *Assessment and Treatment of Articulation and Phonological Disorders* in the *Manual*.

HOW TO USE THE ACCOMPANYING CD-ROM

The CD-ROM that accompanies the *Manual* contains all the printable forms and materials in both Microsoft Word and PDF formats. As already stated in the preface, the Word forms are fully modifiable without any need for copyright permission; the clinician can adapt them to meet his or her professional needs and the child's individual clinical needs. For example, the clinician can personalize the various assessment forms and treatment recording sheets by typing the name of the school or clinic, his or her own name, date, the child's name, and such other personal information typically included on a form that is placed in a student file. The clinician may also delete or add target exemplars from the given word lists, convert target words into phrases and sentences as the child moves through the treatment sequence, alter and personalize letters directed to parents and teachers, and reformat the style of charts and tables if desired.

When the CD is inserted into the computer's CD-ROM drive, the clinician will see two folders—one for the printable PDF forms and one for the modifiable Word forms. Within each folder are separate unit folders. Within each unit folder are form titles. By clicking on the unit folder name (e.g., *Part II: Assessment Resources*), the clinician can see the names of all the files within that folder (e.g., *Nonstandardized Articulation Screening Form*). Clinicians can open and print the preformatted PDF forms, or they can open, modify, and print the Word forms. The forms can be printed on the facility's personalized stationary and placed in the clients' folders or charts.

Preface

◆ ◆ ◆ ◆ ◆ ◆ ◆ ◆ ◆ ◆ ◆ ◆ ◆ ◆

The first edition of *Assessment and Treatment of Articulation and Phonological Disorders in Children*, published in 2000, was two-tiered and included both a basic unit that provided a general overview of a topic (most appropriate for undergraduate study) and an advanced unit that highlighted more complicated or theoretical information (most appropriate for graduate study). Another feature of the book was an extensive list of appendixes that provided the user with clinically practical resources such as sound establishment techniques, word and sentence lists for stimulability testing, treatment plans, sample referral letters, and sample diagnostic reports, to name a few.

As we contemplated the second edition of the textbook, it became clear that to accommodate newer information in both the textbook and the materials in the appendixes, it would be necessary to create a new resource manual for the clinician. Pulling the information in the appendix of the textbook made it possible to create a more comprehensive resource manual for clinicians as well as an expanded textbook that included newer theoretical and practical information for academic courses. The need, as we saw it, was for a user-friendly resource manual to accompany the textbook. Thus emerged this new project.

We wrote this new resource manual to give students and clinicians a practical resource for assessing and treating articulation and phonological disorders in children—a resource that would make professional life a bit easier to manage and execute. We have used many of the materials placed in the original textbook's appendixes, but all have been presented in new, user-friendly formats. Our goal was to provide students and practicing clinicians with a compilation of clinically relevant information in one convenient source. All clinical forms may be either photocopied or, better yet, printed directly from the accompanying CD.

Articulation and Phonological Disorders: Assessment and Treatment Resource Manual is divided into three major parts: *Background Information, Assessment Resources*, and *Treatment Resources*. The first part includes resources such as charts on articulation and phonological development that can be shared with teachers and parents, tables on the phonological characteristics of Spanish-influenced English, African American English, and English influenced by the various Asian languages. Also included are the various internet resources that offer information on currently available Web sites on articulation and phonological disorders and related topics.

The second part focuses on resources that can help expedite the assessment process such as a non-standardized articulation screener, a comprehensive child case history form, a consonant cluster screener, an orofacial screener, a stimulability assessment protocol, and several sample diagnostic reports.

The third and final part provides many treatment resources, including a baseline recording sheet, a sampling of written goals and objectives, data recording sheets, sound establishment techniques for all English consonants, sample treatment activities, word lists for all consonants, written minimal word pairs for contrast training of the common phonological processes, an extensive word list for consonantal and syllabic "r" in different vowel contexts, parent and teacher letters, and much more.

In line with our goal of providing user-friendly and practical information, we avoided theoretical discussions, current controversies, lofty speculations, and unnecessary technical jargon. Although we believe these to be important, we saw them as inappropriate for a resource manual of this nature, and we assumed that the user was already familiar with them. Those interested in such information are referred to the *Manual's* accompanying text-book, *Assessment and Treatment of Articulation and Phonological Disorders in Children—Second Edition*. Because the majority of children with articulation and phonological disorders are serviced by the school-based clinician, the information in the *Manual* was tailored for that setting, but is still appropriate for all clinical settings, with some simple modifications.

As mentioned earlier, all of the practical resources included in this *Manual* are also contained in the accompanying CD. The PDF forms may be printed as they appear in the *Manual*, and the Word forms may be modified and printed without any need for copyright permission. For example, various assessment forms and the baseline and treatment record-ing sheets may be personalized by typing the name of the school or the clinic and the client and the clinician identifying information and then printed out to make it consistent with the school or the clinic stationery. As practicing clinicians ourselves, we see this aspect of the *Manual* as extremely valuable, truly practical, and highly efficient. Our hope is that as you incorporate *Articulation and Phonological Disorders: Assessment and Treatment Resource Manual* into your own clinical practice, you will find the resource manual assessment and treatment planning easier as well as efficient.

We would like to thank Jennifer Gonzalez, an excellent student of ours in speech–language pathology at California State University–Fresno, for her help in searching the aggregated databases for current research information on articulation and phonological disorders and in preparing many of the word lists found in this *Manual*. Her help has been invaluable in completing both the textbook revision and the resource manual on time. We also would like to thank Allen Willard, a graduate of our program, for his help in research-ing the sound establishment techniques included in the *Manual* and other aspects of the textbook. We would also like to thank the many undergraduate and graduate students who inspired us to write the original textbook and this new resource manual.

Part I
Background Information

PHONETIC SYMBOLS FOR ENGLISH SOUNDS

Speech–language pathologists typically use the symbols of the *International Phonetic Alphabet* (IPA) to transcribe sound production errors during an articulation and phonological assessment. Such practice allows for a uniform system that decreases misinterpretation of information among professionals. We recommend the clinician use the symbols of the IPA when recording sound errors so that if other speech–language pathologists review his or her protocols, written reports, and other related documents, the information remains unequivocal.

Phonetic Symbols and Allographs for English Sounds includes the IPA symbols for all English consonants, vowels, and diphthongs and their many *allographic* representations (letter and letter combinations). The clinician can use this table for personal review and can provide a copy to a parent or teacher as an easy reference source, particularly to help them decipher reports and other documents that contain IPA symbols as those related to articulation and phonological disorders often do. See the Basic Unit of Chapter 2 in *Assessment and Treatment of Articulation and Phonological Disorders* for more information on this topic.

Phonetic Symbols and Allographs for English Sounds

IPA Sound Symbol	Sample Allographic Representations
Consonants	
b	**b**aby, ra**bb**it
p	**p**an, pe**pp**er, hiccou**gh**
d	**d**o, la**dd**er, begg**ed**, shou**ld**
t	**t**op, a**tt**ack, talk**ed**, dou**bt**, recei**pt**, **Th**omas
g	**g**et, e**gg**, **g**uest, **gh**ost, va**gue**
k	**k**itchen, a**c**tor, a**cc**ustom, **ch**emistry, bouti**que**
m	**m**oon, ha**mm**er, to**mb**, phle**gm**, hy**mn**, psa**lm**
n	**n**ot, di**nn**er, **kn**ow, **gn**at, **pn**eumonia, **mn**emonic
ŋ	bri**ng**, i**nk**, to**ngue**, a**nx**ious
z	**z**oo, bu**zz**er, **x**ylophone, hi**s**, a**s**thma
s	**s**ay, a**ss**assin, **ps**ychiatrist, li**s**ten, **c**ent
v	**v**alentine, sa**vv**y, wi**fe**'s, Ste**ph**en
f	**f**an, a**ff**air, tou**gh**, tele**ph**one, hal**f**
ð	**th**at, ba**the**
θ	too**th**, **th**in
ʒ	mea**sure**, a**z**ure, gara**ge**
ʃ	**sh**ip, **s**ugar, **ch**ef, mi**ss**ion, loca**tion**
h	**h**op, **wh**o
ʤ	**j**ob, ju**dge**, marri**age**, **g**em, exa**gg**erate
ʧ	**ch**urch, ki**tch**en, na**ture**, **c**ello
w	**wh**en, **w**in, **o**ne, **qu**est, **ch**oir
hw	**wh**ich, **wh**ite, **wh**ere (dialectical variations)
j	**y**ellow, hallelu**j**ah, opin**i**on
r	**r**abbit, ma**rr**y, **wr**ite, **rh**yme, Peace Co**rps**
l	**l**adder, ba**ll**, is**l**and, funne**l**
Vowels	
ɑ	**fa**ther, b**ou**ght, m**o**cking
æ	c**a**t, bl**a**st, j**a**ck f**a**mily
e	m**a**te, l**a**ke, vac**a**tion, rel**ay**
ɛ	b**e**tter, **e**lephant, **e**xit, **e**xplain
o	b**oa**t, m**o**st, t**oa**st, t**o**te
ɔ	f**ou**ght, c**au**ght, f**aw**n, t**a**ll, th**o**ng, w**a**nt
u	m**oo**n, s**ui**tcase, tr**ue**
i	h**ea**t, p**ie**ce, m**ee**k

(continued)

IPA Sound Symbol	Sample Allographic Representations
ɪ	**pi**g, **mi**tt, **ji**ngle, **i**gloo
ʊ	c**oo**k, p**u**t, r**oo**kie
ɚ	batt**er**, jok**er**, col**or**, mak**er**
ɝ	p**ur**ple, b**ir**d, d**ir**ty, p**urr**, **ur**gent
ə	**u**ntie, extr**a**
ʌ	c**u**p, **u**nder, **u**p, b**u**tter

Diphthongs

aɪ	p**i**pe, m**y**, m**igh**t, r**i**te
au	c**ow**, h**ou**se, t**ow**n, p**ou**t
ɔɪ	t**oi**l, b**oy**, m**oi**st, l**oi**ter
ju	**u**nited, **u**sed, f**ew**, b**eau**tiful
eɪ	vac**a**tion, t**a**ke, f**a**ce
ou	l**oa**n, thr**o**ne, ph**o**ne

FREQUENCY OF OCCURRENCE FOR ENGLISH CONSONANTS

Not all consonants occur with the same frequency. In spoken English, some consonants are used often, while others are used very seldom. This is clinically relevant because articulation and phonological errors on frequently occurring sounds may have a greater impact on a child's speech intelligibility and overall communication. For example, a child who misarticulates /r/, which is a frequently occurring consonant, may be more difficult to understand and may draw more negative attention than a child who misarticulates /ʤ/, an infrequently occurring sound.

If the child exhibits multiple misarticulations, the clinician could choose sounds that occur more frequently as initial treatment targets with the expectation that remediation of those sounds would have a more positive effect on the child's speech intelligibility. ***Frequency of Occurrence Rank Order for English Consonants*** provides the frequency of occurrence ranking for all English consonants and can serve as a good resource for the clinician when deciding on initial target sounds.

Frequency of Occurrence Rank Order for English Consonants

Consonant	Rank Order of Frequency of Occurrence
n	1st
t	2nd
s	3rd
r	4th
d	5th
m	6th
z	7th
ð	8th
l	9th
k	10th
w	11th
h	12th
b	13th
p	14th
g	15th
f	16th
ŋ	17th
j	18th
v	19th
ʃ	20th
θ	21st
ʤ	22nd
ʧ	23rd
ʒ	24th

Source: Adapted from "Computer-Assisted Natural Process Analysis (NPA): Recent Issues and Data," by L. D. Shriberg and J. Kwiatkowski, 1983, *Seminars in Speech and Language, 4,* pp. 397–406.

MANNER, PLACE, AND VOICING CHARACTERISTICS

English consonants are often categorized and grouped together according to their manner, place, and voicing features. For example, /m/, /n/, and /ŋ/ are grouped according to their manner of production as the *nasal* sounds. Sounds may also be grouped according to their place of articulation and their voicing features. The sounds /t/, /d/, /s/, /z/, /l/, and /n/, for instance, are categorized as *alveolar* sounds because of their shared places of articulation along the alveolar ridge. Sounds produced with vibration of the vocal folds are labeled *voiced sounds,* while those that are produced without vibration of the vocal folds are considered *voiceless.*

Manner, Place, and Voicing Features of English Consonants is an easy reference source for the clinician who may need a quick review. The clinician may also give a printed copy of the table to an interested parent or teacher. See the Basic Unit of Chapter 2 in *Assessment and Treatment of Articulation and Phonological Disorders* for more information on manner, place, and voicing features of consonants.

Manner, Place, and Voicing Features of English Consonants

Sound	Voicing	Manner	Place
NASALS			
m	+	nasal	bilabial
n	+	nasal	alveolar
ŋ	+	nasal	velar
STOPS			
b	+	stop	bilabial
p	−	stop	bilabial
d	+	stop	alveolar
t	−	stop	alveolar
g	+	stop	velar
k	−	stop	velar
FRICATIVES			
z	+	fricative	alveolar
s	−	fricative	alveolar
v	+	fricative	labiodental
f	−	fricative	labiodental
ð	+	fricative	linguadental
θ	−	fricative	linguadental
ʒ	+	fricative	palatal
ʃ	−	fricative	palatal
h	−	fricative	glottal
hw	−	fricative	glottal/bilabial
AFFRICATES			
ʤ	+	affricate	palatal
ʧ	−	affricate	palatal
GLIDES			
w	+	glide	velar/bilabial
j	+	glide	palatal
LIQUIDS			
r	+	liquid, rhotic*	palatal
l	+	liquid, lateral*	alveolar

*Distinctive feature term

PHONOLOGICAL PROCESSES

Professionals frequently use the term *phonological process* to describe the patterned modifications of the target adult pronunciations found in typically developing children. For example, a 3-year-old child who has not yet acquired many fricatives may substitute stops for those sounds, a phonological process known as *stopping*. Clinically, this term is also used to describe the sound error patterns used by children diagnosed with a phonological disorder.

The occurrence of phonological patterns is common and natural in all children. However, some children continue to demonstrate such patterns beyond the expected age of development. Other children may show patterns that are not common in natural speech development or are unique to the child. These are often called *idiosyncratic processes*.

The clinician may refer to **Definitions and Developmental Data for Common Phonological Processes** for a definition of the most commonly observed phonological processes and the age at which they are expected to disappear. The information on expected ages of disappearance may prove useful to the clinician in deciding whether a specific phonological pattern observed in a child is within normal developmental expectations or not, being cautious to consider individual variability. Refer to the Basic Unit of Chapter 2 in *Assessment and Treatment of Articulation and Phonological Disorders* for an in-depth review of phonological processes if unfamiliar with this topic.

Definitions and Developmental Data for Common Phonological Processes

Process	Definition	Examples	Age of Disappearance
Reduplication	Repetition of a syllable of a target word. Sometimes called *doubling*.	"ba-ba" for bottle "da-da" for dog "ca-ca" for car	by 2½
Diminutization	Addition of /i/ or sometimes a consonant + /i/ to the target word	"cuppy" for cup "bookie" for book "fofee" for finger	by 3
Final consonant deletion	Omission of final consonants	"ha" for hat "mo" for mom "coa" for coat	by 3
Assimilation	A sound in a word changes to become more like another sound in the word. It can affect place of articulation, manner of production, or voicing.	"mom" for mop "cook" for took "boab" for boat "tot" for toss "den" for ten "pick" for pig	by 3
Velar fronting	Replacement of velars "k, g, ng" with sounds made more anterior, particularly alveolars "t, d, n"	"pat" for pack "doat" for goat "rin" for ring	by 3½
Deaffrication	Replacement of an affricate with a stop or fricative	"tair" for chair "sop" for chop "dump" for jump	by 4
Syllable deletion	Omission of one or more syllables from a multi-syllable word	"mato" for tomato "nana" for banana "key" for monkey	by 4
Cluster reduction	Deletion or substitution of some or all parts of a cluster	"pay" for play "ack" for black "gween" for green "op" for stop	by 5
Stopping	Substitution of stops for fricatives and affricates	"pish" for fish "toap" for soap "dis" for this	by 5
Depalatalization	Substitution of an alveolar fricative or affricate for a palatal affricate	"seck" for check "matses" for matches "dudz" for judge "Shen" for Jen	by 5
Gliding	Substitution of liquids "l, r" by glides "w, y"	"wed" for red "cawot" for carrot "yamb" for lamb	beyond 5

Process	Definition	Examples	Age of Disappearance
Vocalization	Substitution of a vowel for a syllabic liquid, syllabic "-er," or postvocalic liquid	"simpo" for simple "papo" for paper "ca" for car	beyond 5
Backing	Replacement of alveolars and palatals "t, d, s, z, n, sh, ch, dge" by sounds made more posterior, particularly "k, g, ng"	"cop" for top "bike" for bite "kip" for ship	⎯⎯

DEVELOPMENTAL INFORMATION FOR PARENTS AND TEACHERS

Many parents wonder when their child of a certain age should be producing specific sounds. Some may even worry that their child has a speech delay that requires professional attention. Classroom teachers may wonder when a referral to a speech–language pathologist is appropriate. Concerned parents, caregivers, and classroom teachers could benefit from reviewing developmental information on sound acquisition and phonological patterns.

We developed ***Letter to Parents and Teachers on Sound Development*** and ***Letter to Parents and Teachers on Phonological Processes*** for parents and classroom teachers. The clinician could provide a printed copy of either or both letters to a child's parent or classroom teacher as a simple reference guide that might help confirm or appease their concerns.

Letter to Parents and Teachers on Sound Development

Dear Parent or Classroom Teacher,

Parents and classroom teachers often wonder at what age their child or student should produce specific speech sounds. Throughout the years, research has suggested general developmental trends. To diagnose articulation and phonological disorders, trained professionals use this information along with many other variables. The age of acquisition presented here is only an average and should not be used exclusively to determine if a child's production of sounds is developing appropriately. Please consult with a trained speech–language pathologist if you are concerned about your child or student's speech development.

Sound	Key Word	Typical Age of Acquisition
	(As used in …)	(arranged from youngest to oldest)
"h"	hot	3
"w"	water	3
"b"	boat	3
"p"	pie	3
"m"	mask	3
"n"	nose	3½
"ng"	ring	3½
"d"	duck	3½
"y"	yellow	4
"g"	gas	4
"t"	tip	4
"k"	kite	4
"f"	fork	5½
"v"	vine	5½
"th" (voiceless)	thick	7
"th" (voiced)	that	7
"sh"	shoe	7
"ch"	chop	7
"j," "-dge"	jam, badge	7
"l"	lung	7
"r"	rabbit	8
"er"	soccer	8
"s"	sick	9
"z"	zoo	9

Please contact me at _____ if you have any questions or concerns.

Sincerely,

_____

Speech–Language Pathologist

Dear Parents and Classroom Teachers,

You may often hear the term *phonological process* used in reference to children who are difficult to understand or who have multiple speech articulation errors. These children, upon close examination by a trained speech–language pathologist, often demonstrate patterns in their simplification of expected word productions primarily by omitting or substituting sounds and/or syllables. In simple terms, the child makes the adult word easier to produce by leaving out whole syllables or by replacing one sound for another in a patterned fashion.

Phonological processes are specific pattern(s) found in the speech of a child. It is important to realize that the presence of phonological processes is common and natural in all children developing speech and language. However, in some children, often for unknown reasons, certain patterns (processes) continue beyond the expected age of development. Other children may exhibit patterns that are not common in natural speech development or are unique to the child.

The following table lists the most common phonological processes, their definition, specific examples, and the age at which you could expect them to disappear. It is very important to keep in mind that to be considered a process, the child's errors must clearly show a pattern, meaning that they must occur several times in his or her productions. A one-time error that fits the definition does not constitute a phonological process. A speech–language pathologist is trained to identify the difference. Some phonological processes have minimal effect on how well a child is understood, while others may have a significant effect. It is common for children to exhibit several phonological processes at the same time. When this is the case, a child's speech typically is very difficult to understand even by parents and other caregivers. If you are concerned about your child or student's speech development, please consult with a trained speech–language pathologist. The information below is shared with you as a general guideline and should not be used to diagnose your child or student with a phonological disorder.

Process	Definition	Examples	Age of Disappearance
Reduplication	Repetition of a syllable of a target word. Sometimes called *doubling*.	"ba-ba" for bottle "da-da" for dog "ca-ca" for car	by 2½
Diminutization	Addition of /i/ or sometimes a consonant + /i/ to the target word	"cuppy" for cup "bookie" for book "fofee" for finger	by 3

Process	Definition	Examples	Age of Disappearance
Final consonant deletion	Omission of final consonants	"ha" for hat "mo" for mom "coa" for coat	by 3
Assimilation	A sound in a word changes to become more like another sound in the word. It can affect place of articulation, manner of production, or voicing.	"mom" for mop "cook" for took "boab" for boat "tot" for toss "den" for ten "pick" for pig	by 3
Velar fronting	Replacement of velars "k, g, ng" with sounds made more anterior, particularly alveolars "t, d, n"	"pat" for pack "doat" for goat "rin" for ring	by 3½
Deaffrication	Replacement of an affricate with a stop or fricative	"tair" for chair "sop" for chop "dump" for jump	by 4
Syllable deletion	Omission of one or more syllables from a multi-syllable word	"mato" for tomato "nana" for banana "key" for monkey	by 4
Cluster reduction	Deletion or substitution of some or all parts of a cluster	"pay" for play "ack" for black "gween" for green "op" for stop	by 5
Stopping	Substitution of stops for fricatives and affricates	"pish" for fish "toap" for soap "dis" for this	by 5
Depalatalization	Substitution of an alveolar fricative or affricate for a palatal affricate	"seck" for check "matses" for matches "dudz" for judge "Shen" for Jen	by 5
Gliding	Substitution of liquids "l, r" by glides "w, y"	"wed" for red "cawot" for carrot "yamb" for lamb	beyond 5
Vocalization	Substitution of a vowel for a syllabic liquid, syllabic "er," or postvocalic liquid	"simpo" for simple "papo" for paper "ca" for car	beyond 5

(*continued*)

Process	Definition	Examples	Age of Disappearance
Backing	Replacement of alveolars and palatals "t, d, s, z, n, sh, ch, dge" by sounds made more posterior, particularly "k, g, ng"	"cop" for top "bike" for bite "kip" for ship	____

Please contact me at _____ if you have any questions or concerns.

Sincerely,

_____

Speech–Language Pathologist

COMMON SOUND ERRORS

On the road to acquiring adultlike speech and language, it is common for children to make articulation errors in predictable patterns. Depending on the child's age, the errors may either be considered developmental and within normal limits or outside of the normal range. Teachers and parents may notice these errors as they interact with their child or student. Young readers who are still in the process of developing their articulation skills may often "misread" a word containing a specific sound. However, it is important for a parent or teacher to recognize that this may simply be due to an articulation error pattern and not a reading miscue. When teachers and parents are made aware of common sound substitution patterns the child's reading "errors" suddenly seem to make sense.

Common Articulation Errors in Typical Sound Acquisition lists some of the most commonly observed articulation errors in young children. The clinician can give a printed copy to a teacher or parent who may benefit from the information. Phonetic symbols were avoided to maintain the readability of the information.

NASALS "m, n, ng"

- A nasal consonant can be replaced by a non-nasal consonant that is made in the same point of contact along the vocal tract. This pattern is known as *denasalization*. *Example*: "dose" for *nose*.
- The final "n" can be replaced by "m" or "ng." *Example*: "fum" for *fun*.
- The final "ng" can be replaced by "n." *Example*: "brin" for *bring*.

GLIDES "y, w, wh"

- The "w," "y," and "wh" can be omitted. *Example*: "ite" for *white*.
- The "y" sound can be replaced by "w, d, h," or "l." *Example*: "lellow" for *yellow*.

STOPS "p, b, t, d, k, g"

- A voiceless sound that occurs at the beginning of words may be replaced by a voiced sound. This pattern is known as *deaspiration* of initial voiceless stops or *initial-consonant voicing*. *Example*: "gat" for *cat*.
- Initial "k" and "g" can be replaced by "t" and "d." This pattern is more common on initial versus final "k" and "g." *Example*: "tup" for *cup*; "dot" for *got*.
- The stops "p, b, t, d, k," and "g" in the final position can be omitted. This pattern is less common for final "k" and "g" than "p, b, t," and "d." *Example*: "ca" for *cat*.

LIQUIDS "l, r"

- The "l" and "r" sounds can be substituted by "w." *Example*: "wadder" for *ladder*; "wabbit" for *rabbit*.
- Initial "l" and "r" can be omitted. *Example*: "ost" for *lost*; "abbit" for *rabbit*.
- The "l" and "r" sounds can be replaced by a rounded vowel and schwa. *Example*: "hout" for *hurt*; "bow" for *bowl*.
- Final "l" and "r" can be omitted. *Example*: "ca" for *car*; "fa" for *fall*.

FRICATIVES "f, v, th" (voiced and voiceless)

- Initial "f, v," and "th" can be replaced by stops sounds. *Example*: "dive" for *five*; "best" for *vest*; "dem" for *them*.
- "th" can be replaced by "f." *Example*: "fumb" for *thumb*; "fat" for *that*.
- Initial and final "v" can be replaced by "b." *Example*: "bacuum" for *vacuum*; "stobe" for *stove*.

- Fricatives can be replaced by other fricatives, as in "f" for "v" and "f" for "th." *Example*: "fife" for *five* and "maf" for *math*.
- Initial "th" can be substituted by fricative "s" or "f." *Example*: "sin" for *thin*; "fink" for *think*.
- Voiceless "th" can be replaced by "f" and voiced "th" can be replaced by "d." *Examples*: "fink" for *think*; "dose" for *those*.

ALVEOLAR PALATAL AFFRICATES AND FRICATIVES "s, z, sh, ch, j/-dge, zh"

- Final "s, z," and "sh" can be omitted. *Example*: "bu" for *bus*; "fi" for *fish*.
- Very young children often replace initial fricatives and affricates with stop sounds (p, b, t, d, k, or g). *Example*: "doo" for *zoo*; "pie" for *five*; "tip" for *ship*.
- Final "z" and "-dge" may be devoiced (that is replaced with a sound that does not have any voicing such as "s" and "ch"). This pattern can also affect initial "z." *Example*: "batch" for *badge*; "soo" for *zoo*.
- Initial and final "sh," "ch," and "dge" can be replaced by sounds that are not made on the hard palate. This is called *depalatalization*. *Example*: "soot" for *shoot*, "tsain" for *chain*, and "ridz" for *ridge*.
- Initial "s" can be replaced by a stop consonant (p, b, t, d, k, or g). *Example*: "toe" for *sew*, "dack" for *sack*, and "pit" for *sit*.
- The "s" sound is often distorted by being made further forward in the mouth or it can be replaced by voiced and voiceless "th." This is commonly known as *lisping*. Examples: "thoap" for *soap*; "thick" for *sick*; "thoup" for *soup*.

DIALECTICAL DIFFERENCES

Considering the pluralism and linguistic diversity within the United States, it is common for the speech–language pathologist to work with children who are culturally and/or linguistically diverse. When assessing or treating a child who is bilingual or speaks in a non-mainstream dialect, the clinician is legally and professionally obligated to consider cultural and linguistic factors in her decision making and service delivery.

We developed *Articulation and Phonological Characteristics of African American English (AAE)*, *Articulation and Phonological Characteristics of Spanish-Influenced English* and *Articulation and Phonological Characteristics of English Influenced by Asian Languages* to provide the clinician with information on the articulation and phonological characteristics of African American English (AAE), Spanish-influenced English, and English influenced by the various Asian languages. The clinician may print and refer to this information while working with children of varied backgrounds. A copy of the tables may also be given to the classroom teacher as a reference guide to help them distinguish a dialectical difference versus a potential articulation or phonological disorder that may warrant referral to a specialist.

See the Basic and Advanced Units of Chapter 5 in *Assessment and Treatment of Articulation and Phonological Disorders* for a detailed review of ethnocultural variables of articulation and phonological development, as well as treatment and assessment considerations.

Articulation and Phonological Characteristics of African American English (AAE)

AAE Articulation and Phonological Features	Mainstream American English (MAE) Production	African American English Counterpart
"l" sound is lessened or omitted	tool	too'
"r" sound is lessened or omitted	door mother protect	doah mudah p'otek
Voiceless "th" is replaced by "f" at the end or in the middle of words	teeth both nothing	teef bof nufin'
Voiceless "th" is replaced by "t" in the beginning of words	think thin	tink tin
Voiced "th" is replaced by "d" in the beginning or in the middle of words	this brother	dis broduh
Voiced "th" is replaced by "v" at the end of words	breathe smooth	breave smoov
Consonant clusters are reduced at the beginning and end of words	throw desk rest wasp	thow des' res' was'
Consonants within clusters are replaced by other consonants	shred strike	sred skrik
Stress patterns of AAE differ from those of MAE	gui**tar** po**lice** Ju**ly**	**gui**tar **po**lice **Ju**ly
Some sounds within a word are reversed in order (*metathetic errors*)	ask	aks
Voiced sounds in the final position are made without voicing	bed rug cab	bet ruk cap
Final consonants are omitted	bad good	ba' goo'
"e" vowel is replaced by "i"	pen ten	pin tin
"v" sound is replaced by "b"	valentine vest	balentine bes'
Diphthongs are reduced (*ungliding*)	find oil	fahnd ol
"ng" is replaced by n	walking thing	walkin thin
Unstressed syllables are omitted	about remember	'bout 'member
Verbs that end in "-ked" are modified	walked liked	wah-tid li-tid

Articulation and Phonological Characteristics of Spanish-Influenced English

Articulation Characteristics	Sample English Patterns
"t, d," and "n" may be *dentalized* (tip of the tongue may be placed against the back of the upper middle teeth)	
Voiced final consonants are made without voicing	"Bop" for *Bob*
"v" is replaced by "b"	"bacuum" for *vacuum*
Stop sounds are not aspirated (*gives the impression that the speaker is leaving out the sound because it is said with very little or no release*)	
"ch" is replaced by "sh"	"shair" for *chair*
voiced "th" is replaced by "d" or "z"	"dis" for *this* "zat" for *that*
Voiceless "th" is replaced by *dentalized* "t"	"mat" for *math*
Schwa sound is added to word-initial consonant clusters	"eschool" for *school* "estar" for *star*
Many final consonants are omitted (in Spanish, words can only end in 10 different sounds: a, e, i, o, u, l, r, n, s, d)	"go" for *got*
Intial "h" may be omitted (*in Spanish the written symbol "h" is silent*)	"elicopter" for *helicopter*
"r" is tapped or trilled (rolled); tapped "r" sounds close to the tap in the English word bu**tt**er	
"j," "-dge" (as in *ju**dge***) is replaced by "y" (*there is no "j"/"-dge" sound in Spanish*)	"yam" for *jam*
"s" sound is made more forward in the mouth closer to the front teeth	some speakers may sound like they have a frontal lisp
Vowels may be substituted and distorted: "i" is replaced by "ee"; "a" is replaced by "e"; "a" is replaced by "ah" (*Spanish only has 5 pure vowels: a, e, i, o, u [ah, e, ee, o, oo] and a few diphthongs*)	"peeg" for *pig* "pet" for *Pat* "Stahn" for *Stan*
"ch" and "sh" confusion (*at times "ch" is replaced by "sh" and at other times "sh" is replaced by "ch"*)	"shair" for *chair* "chef" for *chef* (phonetically speaking)

Articulation and Phonological Characteristics of English Influenced by Asian Languages

Articulation Characteristics	Sample English Productions
Final consonants may be deleted (*in many Asian languages, words end in vowels or just a few consonants*)	"ste" for *step*; "li" for *lid*
Polysyllabic words may be truncated (shortened) or the wrong syllable may be emphasized (*some Asian languages are monosyllabic*)	"ephant" for *elephant*
Voiced consonants may be produced without voicing, particularly those that have a voiceless counterpart (*cognate*)	"luff" for *love*; "pick" for *pig*; "crip" for *crib*; "beece" for *bees*
"r" and "l" confusion (*at times "r" is replaced by "l" and vice a versa*)	"lize" for *rise*; "raundry" for *laundry*
"r" sound may be deleted	"gull" for *girl*; "tone" for *torn*
The vowel in words may be shortened or reduced in length	Vowels sound distorted and words sound "choppy" to English speakers
Voiced and voiceless "th" may be replaced by another sound (*voiced and voiceless "th" do not exist in Asian languages*)	"dose" for *those*; "tin" for *thin*; "zose" for *those*; "sin" for *thin*
Addition of the "uh" sound (*schwa*) in blends or at the end of words (*epenthesis*)	"bulack" for *black*; "wooduh" for *wood*
"ch" and "sh" confusion at times	"sheep" for *cheap*
"a" is replaced by "ah" (*"a" does not exist in many Asian languages*)	"block" for *black*; "shock" for *shack*
"v" is replaced by "b"	"base" for *vase*; "Beberly" for *Beverly*
"w" is replaced by "v"	"vork" for *work*; "vall" for *wall*
"f" is replaced by "p"	"pall" for *fall*; "plower" for *flower*

THE INTERNET AS A VALUABLE RESOURCE

In recent years, the Internet has become a widely used information resource. Individuals can now quickly research any topic of interest out of the comfort of their own home or office. This is no different for the speech–language pathologist or consumers of speech–language services. Currently, there are several sites that provide useful and practical information about communication disorders to individuals, parents, caregivers, and professionals.

We developed ***Web Sites on Articulation and Phonological Disorders and Related Topics*** to simplify the speech–language pathologist's job when researching the many online resources on articulation and phonological disorders. Although not all-inclusive, the Web sites compiled into a useful resource guide are most relevant, practical, parent-friendly, and informative. The clinician or the consumer should search the Web for other or more recently developed sites. We encourage the clinician to print and share the resource guide with parents or classroom teachers who have access to the Internet and who demonstrate an interest in expanding their knowledge of articulation and phonological or other communication disorders.

At the time that this resource manual was published, the following Web sites included a variety of resources for speech–language pathologists, paraprofessionals, and parents. Some Web sites focused on articulation and phonological disorders, while many others included information on a variety of speech, language, and learning disorders.

- **www.slpsite.com** This site, which is listed as a reference on many other Web sites, contains a wealth of information for parents, students, and professionals interested in communication disorders, including articulation and phonological disorders. It is extremely thorough and up-to-date. For ease of navigation, users can browse for information using the table of contents, URL page, or the index.

- **www.speechtx.com** This site has a variety of free printable activities to practice "s," "r," "l," "k," "g," "f," and "sh" in all positions plus final consonant deletion. It also offers some game ideas to incorporate into therapy and makes suggestions regarding books to use for phonological and phonemic awareness training.

- **www.speechteach.co.uk** This site provides speech therapy resources for professionals and parents who assist children with speech and learning difficulties. There are many useful teaching ideas in the resource section, which includes clip art, worksheets, flashcards, games, crafts, parent information, and other teaching aids. Most of this information is downloadable and free.

- **www.members.tripod.com/Freida_vanStaden/SLP.htm** This site is useful for both parents and professionals. It provides many resources for phonemic/phonological awareness, early reading practice, and articulation skills. It includes printable word lists, stories, worksheets, games, and more.

- **www.communicationconnects.com** This Web site is dedicated to providing practical and user-friendly information for speech–language pathologists, teachers, and parents. It provides printable forms, therapy ideas for speech–language pathologists, classroom tips for teachers, home practice ideas and activities for parents, and many other practical resources. The site is easy to navigate and provides links to other related sites.

- **www.angelfire.com/nm2/speechtherapyideas** This Web site was developed as a therapy activity resource for new speech–language pathologists and speech therapy assistants. The site contains information on a variety of communication disorders, including articulation and phonological disorders. It provides links to other speech–language pathology Web sites.

- **http://home.comcast.net/~speechguide/index.html** This site is a source of general information and therapy ideas for apraxia, articulation, augmentative-assisted communication, voice, fluency, language, dysarthria, aphasia, alaryngeal speech, and more. This site was designed for speech–language

(*continued*)

pathologists, professionals in related fields, parents and families, and students. It provides links to journals and articles, products, national and state organizations, departments of education, continuing education and employment resources, and much more.

- **www.apraxia-kids.org** This site contains comprehensive information about childhood apraxia of speech. There are many informative links on getting advice, related articles, upcoming events, current research, available resources, and much more.
- **http://aac.unl.edu/vbstudy.html** This site is intended as a resource for professionals working with children and adults needing an augmentative-alternative mode of communication (AAC). It provides lists of functional vocabulary words and phrases for specific age groups.
- **www.cleftline.org** This Web site of the Cleft Palate Foundation has information related to cleft lip and palate for patients, their families, and health care professionals. The information is available in English and Spanish. In addition to providing useful tips and information about cleft palate, the site has various links to related resources.
- **www.deaflinx.com** This Web site is dedicated to providing factual information and resources related to Deafness and the Deaf culture. In addition to the many links dedicated to the issue of Deafness, there are several useful links for speech-language pathologists including information on oralism, cochlear implants, and cued speech.
- **www.rhymezone.com** This site is an excellent resource for word rhymes, synonyms, antonyms, definitions, and more. Other features on this site include Shakespeare's works, quizzes, famous quotes, nursery rhymes, and famous documents. Clinicians can be creative in how they incorporate the resources on this site in their therapy activities.
- **www.speech-express.com** This site is intended as a resource for parents of young children and teens who struggle with speech, language, and/or communication. Speech–language pathologists and related professionals would find this site to be a valuable resource in their own practice or as a recommendation to parents and teachers. The site offers answers to frequently asked questions, provides information about self-advocacy, offers assistance with homework and tests, and also has an online shop for additional products. It offers information on a variety of communication disorders, including apraxia of speech, dysarthria, and articulation and phonological disorders. A useful feature of this site for articulation and phonological disorders is a list of children's books that target specific sounds, which is conveniently organized according to individual sounds.
- **www.onelook.com** This Web site is a dictionary search engine that uses 970 dictionaries to assist with locating words. Included in the search options are wildcard searching, reverse dictionary look up, pronunciation guides, and translations into many other languages.

- **www.merriamwebster.com** This site offers word searches using a standard dictionary, thesaurus, and child's dictionary for free. Other searches can be performed using collegiate or unabridged versions, and the Encyclopedia Britannica for a membership fee. One of the valuable features of this site is that as a word search is generated, it provides the word's definition(s), pronunciation(s), function, and etymology. An audio icon can be clicked to hear how the word is pronounced.

- **http://www.ed.gov/parents/needs/speced/iepguide/index.html** This section of the U.S. Department of Education Web site offers a guide to the Individualized Education Program (IEP) process for parents, educators, and other agencies. The information provides a full explanation of the IEP process, with examples and links to additional resources.

- **http://bygosh.com/index.html** This site offers free, online literature including novels, nonfiction stories, poems, and children's classics. The owner of the site indicates that all of the free literature featured is no longer under copyright in the United States. The clinician can be creative in how this resource is utilized. Some possibilities include using stories for screening articulation disorders, sound production practice in connected speech, and homework assignments.

- **http://www.magickeys.com/books/index.html** This site offers free, online storybooks for young children, older children, and young adults. The storybooks are beautifully illustrated and the reader can navigate from one page to the next by using the "Next" or arrow icon. Readability scores are provided for each story according to Flesch-Kincaid Grade Level, Flesch Reading Ease, and Gunning Fog Index. The clinician can be creative in how this resource is utilized. Some possibilities include using stories for screening articulation disorders, sound production practice in connected speech, and homework assignments.

- **http://www.wcbdd.org/language_guides.htm** This Web site by the Washington County Board of Developmental Disabilities provides a user-friendly chart outlining the age at which many English consonants can be expected to be produced correctly. It also provides a percentage range of speech intelligibility from ages 18 to 36 months and outlines some general language developmental milestones from birth to 36 months.

- **http://www.helpforkidspeech.org/questions/index.cfm** This Web site, sponsored by the Scottish Rite Foundation of Florida, was developed to help parents and professionals provide better services to children with communication disorders. The Web site provides articles for parents on a variety of issues related to speech, language, learning, and feeding disorders. It also provides a question and answer page that posts answers to selected questions from parents and other interested parties. The site provides a multitude of links to related Web sites. The section on speech sounds under

(continued)

the articles page provides target words and activities for a selected group of sounds. Speech–language pathologists may refer parents to this page for ideas of activities to do at home.

- **http://www.herring.org/speech.html** This Web site provides a vast array of links to information on speech–language pathology. The links are organized into specific categories: Organizations and Associations, General Information, Children, Autism, Augmentative Alternative Communication, Anatomy and Physiology, Neurological Disorders, Voice, Dysphagia, Aphasia, Otolaryngology, Accent Reduction, American Sign Language, Computers and Technology, Publications, and so forth.

Part II
Assessment Resources

CONDUCTING NONSTANDARDIZED SCREENINGS

Before performing or recommending a full articulation and phonological assessment, the clinician may screen the child's skills with standardized or nonstandardized tools. Such tests as the *Test of Minimal Articulation Competence: Rapid Screening Test* (Secord 1981) and *Quick Screen of Phonology* (Bankson & Bernthal 1990) are examples of commercially available standardized screening instruments.

In a nonstandardized articulation and phonological screening, the clinician often engages the child in brief conversation or designs specific questions that help evoke spontaneous verbal productions to record any articulation or phonological errors. The older child with appropriate reading skills may be asked to read a passage while the clinician listens for error productions. The following Web sites provide many stories that can be used during an oral reading screening: http://bygosh.com/index.html and www.magickeys.com/books/index.html. The latter gives a grade-level and readability score for each story.

The clinician can use ***Nonstandardized Articulation Screening Form*** to conduct a nonstandardized speech screening and can use ***Results of Articulation and Phonological Screening Summary Page*** to summarize the results. See the "Basic Unit" of Chapter 2 in *Assessment and Treatment of Articulation and Phonological Disorders* for more detailed information on articulation and phonological screenings.

Nonstandardized Articulation Screening Form

Name: _____

Date of birth: _____

Age: _____

Grade: _____

Referred by: _____

Reason for referral: _____

Date of screening: _____

CONNECTED SPEECH PRODUCTIONS

(List all errors noted on the space provided after each question)

- Tell me your name. _____
- What is your mommy's (daddy's) name? Tell me about your mommy and daddy. _____
_____
- Tell me about your favorite TV show. Who is your favorite person in that show? Why?
_____
- Tell me about your best friend. What kinds of games do you like to play with him
(her)? _____
- Tell me about your favorite cartoon. _____
- Tell me about the last movie you saw. _____
- Tell me what you had for breakfast this morning (or lunch this afternoon). _____
_____
- Tell me about your favorite vacation trip. _____
- Tell me about some presents that you have gotten. Which one is your favorite? Why?
_____
- Say your ABCs. _____
- Count to 20. _____
- Say the days of the week and months of the year. _____
- Sing "Happy Birthday to You." _____

SINGLE-WORD PRODUCTIONS

Instruct the child: "Repeat these words after me."

Record responses as (+) = correct or (−) = incorrect. You may also record the entire production for each word on the space provided. Use the accompanying written word cue cards with children who have appropriate reading skills.

	Initial		Medial		Final	
/p/	pie	_____	apple	_____	lip	_____
/b/	boy	_____	Abby	_____	tub	_____
/t/	ten	_____	mitten	_____	pot	_____
/d/	duck	_____	body	_____	bed	_____
/k/	cut	_____	bucket	_____	sick	_____
/g/	gate	_____	bigger	_____	bug	_____
/f/	fig	_____	muffin	_____	loaf	_____
/v/	van	_____	beaver	_____	hive	_____
/θ/	thought	_____	toothless	_____	math	_____
/ð/	this	_____	bother	_____	bathe	_____
/s/	soap	_____	castle	_____	bus	_____
/z/	zoo	_____	dessert	_____	cheese	_____
/ʃ/	shoe	_____	fishing	_____	dish	_____
/ʒ/			measure	_____	beige	_____
/ʧ/	chop	_____	statue	_____	peach	_____
/ʤ/	juice	_____	pages	_____	badge	_____
/l/	lawn	_____	belly	_____	doll	_____
/r/	rock	_____	carrot	_____	pear	_____
/w/	white	_____	awake	_____		
/j/	yawn	_____	yo-yo	_____		
/ɚ/			bakery	_____	tiger	_____
/ɝ/	earth	_____	bird	_____		

ORAL READING

Passage used: _____

Errors noted: _____

_____

_____

NOTES AND RECOMMENDATIONS

_____

_____

_____

_____

/p/

pie

apple

lip

/b/

boy

Abby

tub

/t/

ten

mitten

pot

/d/

duck

body

bed

/k/

cut

bucket

sick

/g/

gate

bigger

bug

/f/

fig

muffin

loaf

/v/

van

beaver

hive

/θ/

thought

toothless

math

/ð/

this

bother

bathe

/s/

soap

castle

bus

/z/

zoo

dessert

cheese

/ʃ/

shoe

fishing

dish

/ʒ/

_ _ _ _ _

measure

beige

/tʃ/

chop

statue

peach

/dʒ/

juice

pages

badge

/l/

lawn

belly

doll

/r/

rock

carrot

pear

/w/

white

awake

_____

/j/

yawn

yo-yo

_____

/ɚ/

_____

bakery

tiger

/ɝ/

earth

bird

_____

Results of Articulation and Phonological Screening Summary Page

Name: _____

Date of birth: _____

Age: _____

Grade: _____

Teacher: _____

Referred by: _____

Reason for referral: _____

Teacher Reports

Parent Reports

Review of Records

Classroom Observation(s)

Screening Measures
(e.g., interview, reading passage, single words, formal screening test)

Clinical Impressions and Recommendations

_____

Speech–Language Pathologist

GATHERING A CASE HISTORY

A detailed case history is essential in completing a comprehensive speech and language evaluation. A thorough case history can be gathered by (a) collecting a written case history, (b) reviewing reports written by other professionals, and (c) conducting oral interviews with the child's parents. Important factors that may contribute to the articulation or phonological disorder (e.g., history of recurrent ear infections, repaired cleft palate, or familial speech and language delay) may come to light through this process.

In the public school setting, it can sometimes be difficult to collect a case history by interviewing the parents in person. The clinician may need to call the child's home to collect the necessary information or e-mail the child's parents, if appropriate. The clinician may also mail or send a written case history home with the child to be completed by his or her parents.

The clinician may use ***Speech and Language Child Case History Form*** to collect information of the child's communication skills to ensure that important background information does not go unidentified. The clinician may mail the form, send it home with the child for completion by the child's parents, fill it out during a phone interview with the child's parents, or e-mail it as an attachment for the parents to complete and return. See the "Basic Unit" of Chapter 6 in *Assessment and Treatment of Articulation and Phonological Disorders* for more information on gathering a case history.

Speech and Language Child Case History Form

Name: _____

Date of birth: _____

Age: _____

Grade: _____

Teacher: _____

Referred by: _____

Reason for referral: _____

INSTRUCTIONS

Dear Parent(s): Please complete this form to the best of your ability. The responses you provide will help me in the assessment of your child's speech and language skills. The information will be used for diagnostic and treatment purposes only and will not be shared with uninterested parties. Please be assured that your family's confidentiality will be protected.

EARLY SPEECH AND LANGUAGE MILESTONES

- Thinking of your child as an infant, was he or she a quiet or vocal infant? _____
- At what age did your child begin to babble? _____
- At what age did your child begin to imitate your sounds? _____
- At what age did your child say his or her first word? _____
- At what age did your child begin to name people and objects? _____
- At what age did your child begin to put words together (e.g., "Mommy up")? _____
- Were your child's first words and phrases easy or difficult to understand? _____

CURRENT COMMUNICATION STATUS

- At this point, does your child primarily use words or gestures to communicate? _____
- At this point, does your child's speech sound better than it did 6 months ago? _____
- Is your child aware of any speech or communication difficulties? _____
  If yes, how does he or she show this awareness? _____
- What things have you already tried to help your child speak or communicate better?
  _____
  _____
- What have other professionals done to help your child speak or communicate better?
  _____
  _____

- How old was your child when it was first suspected that he or she had a speech or language problem? _____ Who was the first person to notice the problem? _____
- On a range from not a problem to profound (not a problem, mild, moderate, severe, profound), how severe would you judge your child's speech difficulties? _____
- On a scale of 0 to 100, how understandable would you judge your child's speech? _____
- On a scale of 0 to 100, how understandable do you think your child's speech is to strangers or people who are not frequently around him or her? _____
- Have family members or others called negative attention to your child's speech? ___ If so, in what way? _____
- How does your child react to this negative attention? _____

HISTORY OF PROFESSIONAL INTERVENTION

- Has your child's speech and language been evaluated in the past? _____ If so, when and by whom?

  _____

  _____

  What were the results of the evaluation? _____
  Do you have a copy of the report(s)? _____

- Has your child ever received speech treatment? _____ If so, when, for how long, for what reason, and with what degree of success? _____

  _____

  Who was the clinician? _____

- Has your child ever received any other types of services? (e.g., audiological evaluation, specialized dental or orthodontic care, or ENT evaluation) _____
  If yes, when and for what reason?

  _____

  Who was the professional who provided the care?

  _____

  Do you have a copy of any report(s)? _____

HISTORY OF PREGNANCY AND DELIVERY

- Did you (the mother) have any illnesses, accidents, or complications while pregnant with your child? _____

- Did you take any medications while pregnant with your child? _____
- What was the length of your pregnancy with your child? _____
- What was your child's birth weight? _____
- Did your child suffer any complications or unusual conditions at birth or shortly thereafter? _____

CURRENT MEDICAL STATUS AND MEDICAL HISTORY

- What diseases or serious injuries has your child had? _____
  Were there any complications? _____
- Has your child ever been hospitalized? _____
  Please explain. _____
- What is the present condition of your child's health? _____
- Is your child currently receiving any special medications? _____
  Please explain. _____

ACADEMIC AND SOCIAL HISTORY

- If your child attends preschool or elementary school, have his or her teachers reported any difficulties understanding your child's speech or with his or her ability to communicate? _____ Please explain. _____
- What kind of grades or test scores does your child typically receive? _____
  Have his or her teachers reported any learning difficulties?_____
  _____
  Please explain. _____
- Has your child ever been retained a grade in school? _____
- How does your child feel about school and his or her friends and teachers? _____
  _____
- Has your child ever received special academic services or instruction? _____
  Please explain. _____

SOCIAL AND FAMILY HISTORY

- How does your child interact with other children? _____
- How does your child interact with adults? _____
- How does your child get along with others at home? _____

- Do you have other children? _____ If yes, what are their names and ages? _____
  _____
  _____

- What interests, hobbies, or other activities does your child have? _____
  _____

- What are your and your spouse's occupations? _____
  _____

- Please indicate any other information that might help me better understand your concerns about your child's speech and language development.
  _____
  _____
  _____
  _____

- Please indicate the skills you would like your child to achieve through the speech and language program to help him/her communicate better at home, school, and other environments.
  _____
  _____
  _____
  _____

Signature of person completing the form: _____

Relationship to the child: _____

Date form was completed: _____

Thank you in advance for completing this form. If you have any questions or concerns, please call me at _____ or e-mail me at _____ _____. I look forward to working with your child.

_____

Speech–Language Pathologist

CONDUCTING AN OROFACIAL EXAMINATION

Examination of the orofacial structures is necessary to identify any structural problems that may contribute to an articulation disorder. Some articulation disorders are correlated with abnormal structure and function of the orofacial complex. For example, a child with a severe open bite may also have a frontal lisp, a child with a repaired cleft palate may have hypernasal speech, and a child with limited range of movement of the articulators may show distorted or imprecise production of sounds and poor speech intelligibility. We strongly recommend that when assessing a child who has a potential articulation and phonological problem the clinician perform a thorough examination of the speech structures and make appropriate outside referrals if warranted.

The clinician may use ***Orofacial Examination Form*** as a general examination that can help identify some potential problems requiring further assessment by the clinician or related professionals. See the "Basic Unit" of Chapter 6 in *Assessment and Treatment of Articulation and Phonological Disorders* for more information on orofacial examinations.

Name: _____

Date of birth: _____

Age: _____

Grade: _____

Teacher: _____

Referred by: _____

Reason for referral: _____

Date of exam: _____

(Items checked "YES" require closer examination and further evaluation by clinician or other specialists)

STRUCTURE AND FUNCTION OF THE FACIAL MUSCLES

What to look for
→ General symmetry of the face at rest
Questions to consider

- Is there drooping at the corner of the mouth?   Yes _____ No _____
- Is an eyelid partially or completely closed?   Yes _____ No _____
- Is the mandible, or jaw, drooping on one side?   Yes _____ No _____
- Are there any abnormal movements (e.g., facial grimaces, spasms, twitching, etc.)?   Yes _____ No _____
- Are there any signs of mouth breathing or drooling?   Yes _____ No _____

What to look for
→ Symmetry of face while making specific movements
Tasks and questions to consider

- **Ask the child to smile.** Does the corner of the mouth deviate to one side?   Yes _____ No _____
- **Ask the child to open mouth wide.** Does the jaw deviate to one side?   Yes _____ No _____
- **Ask the child to raise both eyebrows.** Do the eyebrows rise evenly?   Yes _____ No _____
- **Ask the child to close the eyes tightly.** Do both eyes close evenly?   Yes _____ No _____

STRUCTURE AND FUNCTION OF THE LIPS

What to look for
→ Structural integrity of the lips
Questions to consider

- Is there drooping at the corner of the mouth? Yes _____ No _____
- Is there an adequate amount of tissue in the lips? Yes _____ No _____
- Do the lips remain closed or apart while at rest? Yes _____ No _____
- Are there any signs of mouth breathing or drooling? Yes _____ No _____
- Does the lip tissue appear healthy? Yes _____ No _____
- Is there any evidence of a repaired cleft lip or other scar tissue? Yes _____ No _____

What to look for
→ Functional integrity of the lips
Tasks and questions to consider

- **Ask the child to smile.** Does the corner of the mouth deviate to one side? Yes _____ No _____
- **Ask the child to pucker.** Does the amount of lip puckering favor one side? Yes _____ No _____
- **Ask the child to alternate between a pucker and a smile.** Does the range of motion appear adequate for speech? Yes _____ No _____
- **Ask the child to puff the cheeks and hold air.** Can the child maintain the air in the mouth to at least the count of 5? Yes _____ No _____
  Is any nasal emission perceived or evident when a mirror is placed under the nares? Yes _____ No _____
- **Ask the child to say "ooo-eee-ooo-eee" in alternating fashion.** Does the range of motion and strength of the lips seem appropriate? Yes _____ No _____

STRUCTURE AND FUNCTION OF THE TONGUE

What to look for
→ Structural integrity of the tongue
Questions to consider

- Does the coloration of the tongue appear normal? Yes _____ No _____
- Does the size of the tongue appear appropriate in relation to the child's oral cavity? Yes _____ No _____

- Are there any signs of atrophy (muscle loss)   Yes _____ No _____
- Are there any abnormal movements (e.g., spasms, fasciculations, writhing, twitches, etc.)?   Yes _____ No _____

What to look for
→ Functional integrity of the tongue
Tasks and questions to consider

- **Ask the child to protrude the tongue as far as possible.** Can the child perform that activity without effort?   Yes _____ No _____
  Does the speed and range of motion appear appropriate?   Yes _____ No _____
  Does the tongue deviate to one side on protrusion?   Yes _____ No _____
- **Ask the child to maintain the tongue in a protruded position to at least the count of 5.** Can the child do this without resting the tongue on the lower lip?   Yes _____ No _____
  Does the tongue rest or hang over the lower lip?   Yes _____ No _____
- **While tongue is protruded, ask the child to move the tongue tip up and down, right and left, and finally from side to side as quickly as possible.** Is the range or motion and excursion appropriate?   Yes _____ No _____
  Are there any signs of groping, uncoordinated movement, or weakness?   Yes _____ No _____
- **Ask the child to retract the tongue.** Does the speed and range of motion appear adequate?   Yes _____ No _____
- **Ask the child to open mouth and lift tongue so that the lingual frenulum is observed.** Is there any sign of ankyloglossia (tongue-tie)?   Yes _____ No _____
- **Ask the child to repeat "la-la-la-la."** Does the range of motion, strength, and excursion of the tongue seem appropriate?   Yes _____ No _____
- **Ask the child to repeat "ka-ka-ka-ka."** Does the range of motion, strength, and excursion of the tongue seem appropriate?   Yes _____ No _____
- **Ask the child to repeat "ka-ka-ka-la."** Does the range of motion, strength, and excursion of the tongue seem appropriate?   Yes _____ No _____

STRUCTURE OF THE HARD PALATE

What to look for
→ Structural integrity of the hard palate
Questions to consider

- Does the coloration of the hard palate appear normal along its midline?   Yes _____   No _____
- Does the height and width of the hard palate vault appear within normal range for speech production?   Yes _____   No _____
- Are there any signs of repaired or unrepaired clefts, fistulas, or fissures?   Yes _____   No _____
- Are there any signs of surgical removal of any portion of the hard palate?   Yes _____   No _____
- Are there any prostheses (e.g., dentures, obturators, palatal lifts)?   Yes _____   No _____

SOFT PALATE STRUCTURE AND FUNCTION

What to look for
→ Structural integrity of the soft palate
Questions to consider

- Does coloration of the soft palate appear normal along its midline (normal coloration is white and pink)?   Yes _____   No _____
- Is the uvula bifid?   Yes _____   No _____
- Are there any signs of repaired or unrepaired clefts, fistulas, or fissures?   Yes _____   No _____
- Are there any signs of surgical removal of any portion of the soft palate?   Yes _____   No _____
- Are there any prostheses (e.g., dentures, obturators, palatal lifts)?   Yes _____   No _____
- Does the velum appear symmetrical?   Yes _____   No _____
- Does the length of the velum appear sufficient for adequate posterior movement in velopharyngeal closure?   Yes _____   No _____

What to look for
→ Functional integrity of the soft palate

- **Engage the child in conversation.** Does the child's speech sound hypernasal or hyponasal? Yes _____ No _____
  Are the pressure consonants produced correctly? Yes _____ No _____
  Are there any unusual substitutions such as pharyngeal fricatives and glottal stops for pressure consonants? Yes _____ No _____
- **Ask the child to produce a prolonged "ah."** Does the velum move up and back to meet the pharyngeal wall? Yes _____ No _____
- **Ask the child to make repeated productions of "ah."** Does the velum move up and back to meet the pharyngeal wall? Yes _____ No _____
- **Ask the child to produce isolated sounds, syllables, or words loaded with non-nasal sounds while placing a small mirror under child's nostrils.** Is there any clouding or fogging of the mirror? (It is important to instruct the child not to exhale as the sounds or words are made to rule out normal exhalation as the cause of the mirror fogging.) Yes _____ No _____

TEETH AND OTHER RELATED STRUCTURES

What to look for
→ Integrity of the teeth and dental arches
Tasks and questions to consider

- **Ask the child to open mouth.** Are there any missing teeth? Yes _____ No _____
  Are the teeth jumbled, tilted, or malpositioned? Yes _____ No _____
  Are there full or partial dentures in place? Yes _____ No _____
  Are there dental appliances (such as braces) in place? Yes _____ No _____
- **Ask the child to bite down gently and separate the lips so that the teeth can be observed.**
  What is the molar occlusal relationship?

  Normal occlusion _____
  Neutrocclusion _____
  Distoclussion _____
  Mesioclussion _____

  What is the bite relationship of the teeth?

  Open bite _____
  Overjet _____
  Closebite _____
  Crossbite _____

  What is the general condition of the teeth? (e.g., hygiene, cavities, breaks, etc.) _____

KEY

Normal occlusion = Lower first molar is approximately half a tooth ahead of the upper molar. Very few individuals have a normal occlusion.

Neutroclussion = Upper and lower dental arches are in normal occlusion; however, individual teeth are misaligned, rotated, or jumbled.

Distoclussion = Lower dental arch is too far back in relation to the upper dental arch. This can often be observed when the mouth is closed; the person has a receding chin (commonly referred to as *overbite*).

Mesioclussion = Lower dental arch is too far forward in relation to the upper dental arch. This is also often observed when mouth is closed; person has a protruding chin (commonly referred to as *underbite*)

Open bite = Lack of contact between upper and lower front teeth despite normal occlusion of the first molars. A central space is created.

Overjet = Excessive horizontal distance between the surfaces of the incisors. A normal distance of 1 to 3 mm of the upper central incisors in relation to the lower central incisors can be expected.

Closebite = Excessive vertical overlapping of the upper front teeth over the lower front teeth. The upper front teeth cover more than the usual half to one-third of the lower teeth. Occlusion of the molars is normal.

Crossbite = Lateral overlapping of the upper and lower dental arches. The lower jaw is either to the right or to the left of a normal, central position in relation to the upper jaw.

DIADOCHOKINETIC SYLLABLE RATES

[pʌ-pə-pə] # of repetitions _____ # of seconds _____

[tʌ-tə-tə]   # of repetitions _____ # of seconds _____

[kʌ-kə-kə] # of repetitions _____ # of seconds _____

[fʌ-fə-fə]   # of repetitions _____ # of seconds _____

[lʌ-lə-lə]   # of repetitions _____ # of seconds _____

[pʌ-tə-kə] # of repetitions _____ # of seconds _____

OTHER OBSERVATIONS

_____

_____

_____

OBTAINING DIADOCHOKINETIC SYLLABLE RATES

Diadochokinetic syllable rates refer to the speed and regularity with which a person produces repetitive articulatory movements. They help assess the functional and structural integrity of the lips, jaw, and tongue for rapid repetition of syllables and are most clinically significant in the assessment of such motor speech disorders as apraxia, dysarthria, and other articulation disorders caused by poor oral motor movements. Adults with apraxia of speech and children with childhood apraxia of speech may display significant breakdown in appropriate sequencing of syllables. Adults or children with dysarthria may show irregular, slow, labored, or accelerated yet imprecise syllable rates secondary to muscle weakness, paralysis, or incoordination.

If the clinician suspects that a child's articulation difficulties may be motor-based, it is important that he or she obtains diadochokinetic rates during assessment. The information obtained can both help guide a diagnosis and serve as pretreatment data that can shed light on the child's improvement during treatment. It is clinically wise to make diadochokinetic testing a common practice with severely unintelligible children since the underlying cause of their poor speech intelligibility may be related to motor programming or motor weakness.

The clinician may use **Diadochokinetic Syllable Rates Examination Form** to obtain and record diadochokinetic syllable rates. See the "Basic Unit" of Chapter 6 in *Assessment and Treatment of Articulation and Phonological Disorders* for more information on the assessment and treatment implications of diadochokinetic syllable rates.

Diadochokinetic Syllable Rates Examination Form

Name: _____

Date of birth: _____

Age: _____

Grade: _____

Teacher: _____

Referred by: _____

Reason for referral: _____

Date of exam: _____

_____ *Pretreatment Assessment*

_____ *Posttreatment Assessment*

Instruct the child, *"Please take a deep breath and say _____ as long and as evenly as you can."* Model the response for the child to imitate to avoid misunderstanding of the task. Say, *"Try doing it like me…"*

[pʌ-pə-pə]   # of repetitions _____   # of seconds _____

[tʌ-tə-t ə]   # of repetitions _____   # of seconds _____

[kʌ-kə-kə]   # of repetitions _____   # of seconds _____

[fʌ-fə-f ə]   # of repetitions _____   # of seconds _____

[lʌ-lə-lə]   # of repetitions _____   # of seconds _____

[pʌ-tə-kə]   # of repetitions _____   # of seconds _____

Compare child's performance to developmental data:

Average Number of Seconds

Age	20 reps			15 reps			10 reps		
	pʌ	tʌ	kʌ	fʌ	lʌ	pʌtə	pʌkə	tʌtə	pʌtəkə
6	4.8	4.9	5.5	5.5	5.2	7.3	7.9	7.8	10.3
7	4.8	4.9	5.3	5.4	5.3	7.6	8.0	8.0	10.0
8	4.2	4.4	4.8	4.9	4.6	6.2	7.1	7.2	8.3
9	4.0	4.1	4.6	4.6	4.5	5.9	6.6	6.6	7.7
10	3.7	3.8	4.3	4.2	4.2	5.5	6.4	6.4	7.1
11	3.6	3.6	4.0	4.0	3.8	4.8	5.8	5.8	6.5
12	3.4	3.5	3.9	3.7	3.7	4.7	5.7	5.5	6.4
13	3.3	3.3	3.7	3.6	3.5	4.2	5.1	5.1	5.7

Source: Adapted from Fletcher 1972, 1978.

Clinical Impressions and Recommendations:

_____

_____

_____

ASSESSING CONSONANT CLUSTERS

Children with articulation and phonological disorders often demonstrate difficulties with consonant clusters; however, standardized tests may or may not examine their production or may restrict testing to a selected number of clusters. Standardized tests that include phonological processes generally examine consonant clusters more thoroughly because cluster reduction may be a presenting process; however, the focus may still be on a limited number of clusters.

Initial and Final Consonant Clusters Screening Form can be used as a general screener for the production of initial and final clusters or as a baseline of the child's production of a variety of clusters. Care should be taken in the use of Initial and Final Consonant Clusters Screening Form, as it is not standardized and is provided only as a way of supplementing the clinician's thorough assessment of the child's articulation and phonological skills. Developmental data are provided only for those clusters for which they were available.

Initial and Final Consonant Clusters Screening Form

Name: _____

Date of birth: _____

Age: _____

Grade: _____

Teacher: _____

Referred by: _____

Reason for referral: _____

Date: _____

KEY

✓ = correct production

X = incorrect production

Record error in space provided

Instructions: Tell the child, "Say _____" and provide a clear model of the test word. Record responses. Use the accompanying written word cue cards with children who have appropriate reading skills.

INITIAL CLUSTERS

/kw/	quick _____	queen _____	quack _____	4-0
/tw/	twist _____	twin _____	twenty _____	4-0
/sw/	swim _____	swap _____	sweat _____	7-0
/pl/	play _____	plan _____	plate _____	4-0
/kl/	clock _____	clap _____	clean _____	4-0
/fl/	flat _____	fly _____	fleet _____	5-0
/bl/	blip _____	blame _____	blow _____	4-0
/gl/	glass _____	glad _____	glow _____	4-0
/sl/	sleep _____	slide _____	sly _____	7-0
/pr/	press _____	prize _____	prime _____	4-0
/br/	brag _____	brain _____	brown _____	4-0
/tr/	tree _____	trap _____	trick _____	4-0
/dr/	drip _____	dress _____	dry _____	4-0
/fr/	frog _____	fry _____	frame _____	5-0
/θr/	three _____	throw _____	thrive _____	7-0
/kr/	crop _____	cream _____	cry _____	4-0
/gr/	gray _____	grass _____	grin _____	5-0

/st/	stop	_____	stick	_____	stay	_____	4-0
/sp/	spot	_____	speak	_____	spine	_____	4-0
/sk/	scoop	_____	scout	_____	scone	_____	4-0
/sn/	snake	_____	snow	_____	sniff	_____	4-0
/sm/	smile	_____	smog	_____	smash	_____	4-0
/nj/	new	_____	newt	_____	news	_____	----
/fj/	few	_____	fume	_____	fuel	_____	----
/kj/	cute	_____	Cuba	_____	cube	_____	----
/mj/	muse	_____	music	_____	mute	_____	----
/ʃr/	shrine	_____	shriek	_____	shred	_____	7-0
/str/	straw	_____	stray	_____	street	_____	5-0
/skw/	squat	_____	squeal	_____	squint	_____	6-0
/spl/	splint	_____	splash	_____	split	_____	7-0
/spr/	spray	_____	sprig	_____	spree	_____	7-0
/skr/	scram	_____	scream	_____	scrap	_____	7-0

FINAL CLUSTERS

/mp/	lamp	_____	ramp	_____	jump	_____	4-0
/nt/	hint	_____	ant	_____	count	_____	6-0
/nd/	hand	_____	bend	_____	fond	_____	6-0
/ns/	wince	_____	mince	_____	fence	_____	----
/rd/	hard	_____	lard	_____	gourd	_____	5-0
/nz/	lens	_____	buns	_____	beans	_____	----
/ks/	likes	_____	lacks	_____	wakes	_____	4-0
/st/	past	_____	test	_____	most	_____	7-0
/kt/	act	_____	fact	_____	locked	_____	8-0
/ld/	held	_____	mold	_____	fold	_____	----
/rt/	art	_____	cart	_____	sort	_____	4-0
/ts/	bets	_____	mats	_____	mitts	_____	----
/rn/	torn	_____	warn	_____	barn	_____	5-0
/rm/	arm	_____	farm	_____	dorm	_____	4-0
/lp/	pulp	_____	help	_____	gulp	_____	4-0
/lt/	malt	_____	halt	_____	belt	_____	4-0
/lf/	self	_____	golf	_____	elf	_____	5-0
/lk/	elk	_____	bulk	_____	milk	_____	6-0
/zd/	buzzed	_____	dazed	_____	raised	_____	----
/rk/	park	_____	fork	_____	mark	_____	4-0

/mz/	arms	_____	aims	_____	stems	_____	----
/lz/	balls	_____	malls	_____	sells	_____	----
/gz/	bugs	_____	pigs	_____	begs	_____	----
/pt/	opt	_____	kept	_____	swept	_____	4-0
/ft/	left	_____	soft	_____	lift	_____	4-0
/rf/	scarf	_____	wharf	_____	morph	_____	5-0
/rv/	starve	_____	carve	_____	swerve	_____	----
/mpt/	bumped	_____	stamped	_____	jumped	_____	4-0
/mps/	lamps	_____	ramps	_____	bumps	_____	4-0
/nts/	ants	_____	pants	_____	rants	_____	----
/ŋz/	sings	_____	gongs	_____	kings	_____	----
/ŋk/	thank	_____	bank	_____	junk	_____	4-0
/ndz/	hands	_____	lends	_____	bends	_____	----

Notes and Observations:

_____

_____

_____

_____

/kw-/

quick

queen

quack

/tw-/

twist

twin

twenty

/sw-/

swim

swap

sweat

/pl-/

play

plan

plate

/kl-/

clock

clap

clean

/fl-/

flat

fly

fleet

/bl-/

blip

blame

blow

/gl-/

glass

glad

glow

/sl-/

sleep

slide

sly

/pr-/

press

prize

prime

/br-/

brag

brain

brown

/tr-/

tree

trap

trick

/dr-/

drip

dress

dry

/fr-/

frog

fry

frame

/θr-/

three

throw

thrive

/kr-/

crop

cream

cry

/gr-/

gray

grass

grin

/st-/

stop

stick

stay

/sp-/

spot

speak

spine

/sk-/

scoop

scout

scone

/sn-/

snake

snow

sniff

/sm-/

smile

smog

smash

/nj-/

new

newt

news

/fj-/

few

fume

fuel

/kj-/

cute

Cuba

cube

/mj-/

muse

music

mute

/ʃr-/

shrine

shriek

shred

/str-/

straw

stray

street

/skw-/

squat

squeal

squint

/spl-/

splint

splash

split

/spr-/

spray

sprig

spree

/skr-/

scram

scream

scrap

/-mp/

lamp

ramp

jump

/-nt/

hint

ant

count

/-nd/

hand

bend

fond

/-ns/

wince

mince

fence

/-rd/

hard

lard

gourd

/-nz/

lens

buns

beans

/-ks/

likes

lacks

wakes

/-st/

past

test

most

/-kt/

act

fact

locked

/-ld/

held

mold

fold

/-rt/

art

cart

sort

/-ts/

bets

mats

mitts

/-rn/

torn

warn

barn

/-rm/

arm

farm

dorm

/-lp/

pulp

help

gulp

/-lt/

malt

halt

belt

/-lf/

self

golf

elf

/-lk/

elk

bulk

milk

/-zd/

buzzed

dazed

raised

/-rk/

park

fork

mark

/-mz/

arms

aims

stems

/-lz/

balls

malls

sells

/-gz/

bugs

pigs

begs

/-pt/

opt

kept

swept

/-ft/

left

sift

lift

/-rf/

scarf

wharf

morph

/-rv/

starve

carve

swerve

/-mpt/

bumped

stamped

jumped

/-mps/

lamps

ramps

bumps

/-nts/

ants

pants

rants

/-ŋz/

sings

gongs

kings

/-ŋk/

thank

bank

junk

/-ndz/

hands

lends

bends

PERFORMING A MANNER, PLACE, AND VOICING ANALYSIS OF SOUND ERRORS

One of the most basic types of sound error pattern analyses is the manner, place, and voicing (MPV) method. This type of analysis considers a child's misarticulations in relation to the phonetic features of manner, place, and voicing (see "Printable Manner, Place, and Voicing Features of English Consonants" in this *Resource Manual* for a review of these features). Through this type of analysis, the clinician may discover that a child frequently substitutes alveolar sounds for palatal and velar sounds, which is a problem with *place of articulation*. A pattern that affects the *manner of production* may be observed in a child who substitutes fricatives for stops, or glides for liquids. Multiple substitutions of voiceless for voiced consonants would be described as an error pattern affecting the *voicing feature* of sounds. An MPV analysis may be performed from the information obtained in single-word tests or a connected speech sample. It is not a complicated type of analysis.

After identifying particular substitution patterns, the clinician may choose to teach one or more exemplars of the affected sound class. For example, if velars are frequently replaced by alveolars, the clinician may choose to teach one of the velar sounds within the class and then probe for generalized productions to the untaught sounds. Or, the clinician may choose to teach all velars /k, g,/ and /ŋ/ simultaneously.

Manner, Place, and Voicing Analysis Worksheet allows the clinician to perform an MPV analysis on information gathered from a single-word test and or a connected speech sample. See the "Basic Unit" of Chapter 6 in *Assessment and Treatment of Articulation and Phonological Disorders* for more information on MPV analysis.

Manner, Place, and Voicing Analysis Worksheet

Name: _____

Date of birth: _____

Age: _____

Grade: _____

Teacher: _____

Referred by: _____

Reason for referral: _____

Connected speech: _____

Single words: _____

Formal test: _____

Analysis by Manner of Production

	Produced Correctly (+)	Misarticulated (record specific error)
Nasals		
/m/	_____	_____
/n/	_____	_____
/ŋ/	_____	_____
Stops		
/p/	_____	_____
/b/	_____	_____
/t/	_____	_____
/d/	_____	_____
/k/	_____	_____
/g/	_____	_____
Fricatives		
/f/	_____	_____
/v/	_____	_____
/s/	_____	_____
/z/	_____	_____
/θ/	_____	_____
/ð/	_____	_____
/ʃ/	_____	_____
/ʒ/	_____	_____
/h/	_____	_____
Affricates		
/tʃ/	_____	_____
/dʒ/	_____	_____

Glides

/j/   _____   _____

/w/   _____   _____

Liquids

/l/   _____   _____

/r/   _____   _____

Analysis by Place of Articulation

	Produced Correctly (+)	Misarticulated (record specific error)
Bilabials		
/m/	_____	_____
/b/	_____	_____
/p/	_____	_____
/w/	_____	_____
Alveolars		
/t/	_____	_____
/d/	_____	_____
/s/	_____	_____
/z/	_____	_____
/n/	_____	_____
/l/	_____	_____
Palatals		
/ʃ/	_____	_____
/ʒ/	_____	_____
/tʃ/	_____	_____
/dʒ/	_____	_____
/j/	_____	_____
/r/	_____	_____
Linguadentals		
/θ/	_____	_____
/ð/	_____	_____
Labiodentals		
/f/	_____	_____
/v/	_____	_____
Velars		
/k/	_____	_____
/g/	_____	_____
/ŋ/	_____	_____
Glottals		
/h/	_____	_____

Analysis by Voicing Dimensions

	Produced Correctly (+)	**Misarticulated (record specific error)**
Voiced Consonants		
/m/	_____	_____
/n/	_____	_____
/ŋ/	_____	_____
/b/	_____	_____
/d/	_____	_____
/g/	_____	_____
/v/	_____	_____
/ð/	_____	_____
/z/	_____	_____
/ʒ/	_____	_____
/dʒ/	_____	_____
/r/	_____	_____
/l/	_____	_____
/w/	_____	_____
/j/	_____	_____
Voiceless Consonants		
/p/	_____	_____
/t/	_____	_____
/k/	_____	_____
/f/	_____	_____
/θ/	_____	_____
/s/	_____	_____
/ʃ/	_____	_____
/h/	_____	_____

Clinical impressions: _____

_____

_____

_____

Notes: _____

_____

_____

_____

PERFORMING A PHONOLOGICAL PROCESS ANALYSIS OF WORD PRODUCTION

A current method of analysis in the assessment of phonological disorders is the *phonological process analysis approach*. The child's sound errors are classified according to the phonological processes evident in the child's speech. This type of analysis is most often used with highly unintelligible children who have multiple sound production errors.

Phonological processes can be assessed according to their *frequency of occurrence* and *percentage of occurrence*. A frequency of occurrence would identify the number of times a specific process occurs in a child's speech sample, while percentage of occurrence identifies the number of times a process occurs, plus the percentage with which it occurs. McReynolds and Elbert (1981) suggest that to qualify as a process, an error must have an opportunity to occur in at least four instances in a collected speech sample, and it must occur in a least 20% of those opportunities. Hodson and Paden (1991) offer a more stringent criterion by stating that a phonological process must have at least a 40% occurrence before it is selected as a treatment target.

The clinician may use **Phonological Process Analysis Worksheet** to identify the frequency of occurrence and percentage of occurrence from a collected sample of words. This information may guide the clinician in the selection of phonological processes for remediation. See the "Basic Unit" of Chapter 6 in *Assessment and Treatment of Articulation and Phonological Disorders* for more information on this topic.

Phonological Process Analysis Worksheet

Name: _____

Date of birth: _____

Age: _____

Grade: _____

Teacher: _____

Referred by: _____

Reason for referral: _____

Connected speech: _____

Single words: _____

Formal test: _____

Intended Production	Child's Production	Phonological Pattern(s)
_____	_____	_____
_____	_____	_____
_____	_____	_____
_____	_____	_____
_____	_____	_____
_____	_____	_____
_____	_____	_____
_____	_____	_____
_____	_____	_____
_____	_____	_____
_____	_____	_____
_____	_____	_____
_____	_____	_____
_____	_____	_____
_____	_____	_____
_____	_____	_____
_____	_____	_____
_____	_____	_____
_____	_____	_____
_____	_____	_____

Intended Production	Child's Production	Phonological Pattern(s)
_____	_____	_____
_____	_____	_____
_____	_____	_____
_____	_____	_____
_____	_____	_____
_____	_____	_____
_____	_____	_____
_____	_____	_____
_____	_____	_____
_____	_____	_____
_____	_____	_____
_____	_____	_____
_____	_____	_____
_____	_____	_____
_____	_____	_____
_____	_____	_____
_____	_____	_____
_____	_____	_____
_____	_____	_____
_____	_____	_____
_____	_____	_____
_____	_____	_____
_____	_____	_____
_____	_____	_____
_____	_____	_____
_____	_____	_____
_____	_____	_____
_____	_____	_____
_____	_____	_____
_____	_____	_____
_____	_____	_____
_____	_____	_____
_____	_____	_____
_____	_____	_____

Intended Production	Child's Production	Phonological Pattern(s)
_____	_____	_____
_____	_____	_____
_____	_____	_____
_____	_____	_____
_____	_____	_____
_____	_____	_____
_____	_____	_____
_____	_____	_____
_____	_____	_____
_____	_____	_____
_____	_____	_____
_____	_____	_____

Frequency of occurrence for each process: _____

_____

_____

_____

Percentage of occurrence for each process (# of actual occurrences divided by total # of opportunities for the process to occur): _____

_____

_____

_____

Clinical impressions: _____

_____

_____

COLLECTING A CONNECTED SPEECH SAMPLE

Because the production of sounds in single words may not represent a child's articulation and phonological proficiency in connected speech, it is essential to obtain a sample of connected speech during assessment. This will help obtain a more valid picture of the child's articulation and phonological skills than can be obtained from standardized test results alone. In general, between 100 to 200 words may provide a representative sample, and depending on the child's language proficiency and willingness to talk, between 50 to 150 utterances are usually sufficient to obtain the recommended number of words. Ultimately, the clinician must decide the number of words and utterances needed for a representative sample.

For a child who is extremely resistant to talk in the clinical setting, the clinician may ask the parents to bring in a tape recording of their child's speech and language at home. Depending on the child's level of intelligibility, the clinician may decide to use narrow versus broad phonetic transcription to transcribe the collected sample.

Connected Speech Sample Transcription Recording and Analysis Form can be used to transcribe a connected speech sample. See the "Basic Unit" of Chapter 6 in *Assessment and Treatment of Articulation and Phonological Disorders* for more in-depth information on connected speech and language samples.

Connected Speech Sample Transcription Recording and Analysis Form

Name: _____

Date of birth: _____

Age: _____

Grade: _____

Teacher: _____

Referred by: _____

Reason for referral: _____

Date sample taken: _____

_____

_____

_____

_____

_____

_____

_____

_____

_____

_____

_____

_____

_____

_____

_____

_____

_____

_____

_____

_____

_____

_____

_____

Sample Analysis & Clinical Impressions:
(The following information was obtained from the transcribed connected speech sample):

Specific sound errors:

Patterns in articulation errors:

Phonological processes:

Consistency of error productions:

Errors noted in sample but not in single-word test:

Errors noted in single-word test but not connected speech sample:

Clinical impression of intelligibility:

Other observations:

IDENTIFYING SPEECH INTELLIGIBILITY

Articulation and phonological errors affect a child's speech intelligibility to varying degrees. In some children, the effect may be significant and in others it may be minimal. Children diagnosed with a severe phonological disorder usually are very difficult to understand, while children who have sound-specific phonetic errors may remain 100% understandable despite such errors.

If poor speech intelligibility is a problem, it is important to obtain a *pretreatment* measure of intelligibility to assess the effectiveness of therapy over a period of time. It can be expected that as the child's articulation or phonological skills improve, speech intelligibility will also improve. The clinician may obtain *posttreatment* measures of intelligibility after a specific period of time and compare that with the child's pretreatment level of intelligibility.

When assessing the child's speech intelligibility, the clinician can either use a *rating scale* or calculate *percentage of intelligibility*. **Speech Intelligibility Rating Scales, Objective Methods of Analysis, and Age Expectations** lists some clinical judgment scales of intelligibility and outlines methods for calculating percentages of intelligibility. Developmental ranges of speech intelligibility are also provided to help the clinician compare the child's level of intelligibility with what can be typically expected at varying ages.

RATING SCALES

3-point Clinical Judgment Scale of Intelligibility

1 Very understandable
2 Understandable when the topic is known
3 Not understandable even with careful listening

5-point Clinical Judgment Scale of Intelligibility

1 Understandable all of the time
2 Understandable most of the time
3 Understandable about half the time
4 Not very understandable
5 Not understandable at all

Percentage-Based Clinical Impression of Intelligibility

0%–20% Intelligible	→	Completely unintelligible
20%–40% Intelligible	→	Unintelligible most of the time
40%–60% Intelligible	→	Intelligible about half of the time
60%–80% Intelligible	→	Intelligible about three-quarters of the time
80%–90% Intelligible	→	Intelligible most of the time
90%–100% Intelligible	→	Completely intelligible

OBJECTIVE METHODS OF ANALYSIS

Method 1

Step 1: Collect a connected speech sample. Record the sample for later analysis.

Step 2: Transcribe the sample. Do not make a concerted effort to understand the child as the sample is being transcribed from recording. Write out each word for each utterance. Intelligible words may be written orthographically as opposed to phonetically for this purpose.

Step 3: Use a symbol that helps depict an unintelligible word such as a slash (/) or squiggle mark (~).

Step 4: Calculate intelligibility for words spoken. Divide the total number of intelligible words by the total number of words. For example: 105 intelligible words ÷ 250 total (intelligible + unintelligible) words = 42% intelligibility for words.

Method 2

Step 1: Randomly select 200 consecutive words from the child's tape-recorded contextual speech sample.

Step 2: Play back the recorded sample, listen to the sample, and count the number of *unintelligible words*.

Step 3: Subtract the number of *unintelligible words* from 200 and divide the remaining number by 2.

Step 4: The answer is the intelligibility percentage score for the child. For example: 200 total words − 50 unintelligible words = 150 words / 2 = 75% intelligibility for words (*Note:* Adapted from Weiss, Gordon, & Lillywhite 1987).

SPEECH INTELLIGIBILITY EXPECTATIONS ACCORDING TO AGE RANGE (APPROXIMATES)

18 months	25% intelligible
24 months	50% intelligible
2–3 years	50%–75% intelligible
3–4 years	75%–90% intelligible
5+ years	90%–100% intelligible (a few articulation errors may persist)

PERFORMING STIMULABILITY ASSESSMENT

After a child's articulation and phonological skills have been thoroughly examined, the clinician may test the level of stimulability for some or all of the error sounds. *Stimulability* refers to a child's correct or improved production of a misarticulated sound when given a model or other stimulation (e.g., phonetic placement cues). Some standardized articulation tests such as the *Goldman-Fristoe Test of Articulation* (Goldman & Fristoe 2000) and the *Test of Minimal Articulation Competence* (Secord 1981) offer a section for stimulability testing, while others do not.

Stimulability Assessment in Words and Sentences Protocol provides the clinician with the necessary stimuli to assess stimulability of all English consonants at the sound, word, and sentence levels. With children who have multiple misarticulations, the clinician can limit testing to sounds that are potential therapy targets and can use the corresponding forms.

During stimulability testing, the clinician gains the child's attention, provides an exaggerated model of the target sound, asks the child to imitate the model, and provides positive feedback for the child's efforts. Although there is currently no standard for what type of stimulation should be provided, most examiners minimally assess the child's improved production with the clinician's model; however, other types of stimulation may be provided (listed below from least to maximal level of stimulation):

- Model only: "Joey, listen closely as I say the word <u>c</u>ow. Now you say <u>c</u>ow."
- Model + visual cue: While in front of a mirror, the clinician says, "Joey, look how the back of my tongue touches the roof of my mouth way in the back when I say the word <u>c</u>ow. Now you try putting your tongue back there when you say <u>c</u>ow."
- Model + tactile placement cue: The clinician assists the child's placement of the back of the tongue against the velum with a tongue depressor or other instrument and provides an auditory model. "Joey, when I say the word <u>c</u>ow, my tongue is way in the back as I make the *k* sound. Let me help you make that sound."
- Model + any combination: The clinician provides an auditory model plus a combination of visual, tactile, and phonetic placement cues.

See the "Basic Unit" of Chapter 6 in *Assessment and Treatment of Articulation and Phonological Disorders* for the diagnostic and treatment implications of stimulability testing.

Stimulability Assessment in Words and Sentences Protocol

Name: _____

Age: _____

Date of birth: _____

Grade: _____

Referred by: _____

Date of exam: _____

Articulation Test or Method of Assessment: _____

List the sounds that were produced in error during articulation and phonological assessment:

_____

_____

_____

_____

LEVEL OF STIMULATION KEY

M = Model only

M + V = Model plus visual cue

M + T = Model plus tactile placement cue

M + C = Model plus combination of cues

SOUND

/p/

Initial Position	Results	Level of Stimulation
pot	_____	_____
pan	_____	_____
pad	_____	_____
pipe	_____	_____
pack	_____	_____
I cook in a pot.	_____	_____
The pan is very hot.	_____	_____
The pad is soft.	_____	_____
Bob found a pipe.	_____	_____
Pack your clothes.	_____	_____

Medial Position	Results	Level of Stimulation
happy	_____	_____
copy	_____	_____
apple	_____	_____
open	_____	_____
hippo	_____	_____
The boy is happy.	_____	_____
Give me a copy.	_____	_____
I want an apple.	_____	_____
The door is open.	_____	_____
The hippo is very big.	_____	_____

Final Position	Results	Level of Stimulation
dip	_____	_____
cup	_____	_____
deep	_____	_____
soup	_____	_____
mop	_____	_____
Dip the cone.	_____	_____
I want a cup of tea.	_____	_____
The pool is not deep.	_____	_____
The soup is very hot.	_____	_____
Please mop the floor.	_____	_____

/b/

Initial Position	Results	Level of Stimulation
bag	_____	_____
ball	_____	_____
bee	_____	_____
bike	_____	_____
bed	_____	_____
Take the bag.	_____	_____
The ball is red.	_____	_____
The bee is fast.	_____	_____
I got a new bike.	_____	_____
It is time for bed.	_____	_____

Medial Position	Results	Level of Stimulation
bubble	_____	_____
labor	_____	_____
maybe	_____	_____
Bobby	_____	_____
obey	_____	_____
I like bubble gum.	_____	_____
This is hard labor.	_____	_____
Maybe he will come.	_____	_____
Bobby went home.	_____	_____
Obey your parents.	_____	_____

Final Position	Results	Level of Stimulation
cab	_____	_____
babe	_____	_____
mob	_____	_____
tub	_____	_____
web	_____	_____
Take a cab.	_____	_____
The babe is sick.	_____	_____
The mob is loud.	_____	_____
She is in the tub.	_____	_____
I saw a web.	_____	_____

/t/

Initial Position	Results	Level of Stimulation
tape	_____	_____
tea	_____	_____
tan	_____	_____
ten	_____	_____
Ted	_____	_____
Where is the tape?	_____	_____
May I have some tea?	_____	_____
She has a deep tan.	_____	_____
Lisa can count to ten.	_____	_____
Ted went to the store.	_____	_____

Medial Position	Results	Level of Stimulation
tomato	_____	_____
potato	_____	_____
guitar	_____	_____
hotel	_____	_____
detail	_____	_____
Tomatoes taste good.	_____	_____
I like baked potatoes.	_____	_____
Can you play the guitar?	_____	_____
He stayed in a hotel.	_____	_____
Please tell me the details.	_____	_____

Final Position	Results	Level of Stimulation
bait	_____	_____
ate	_____	_____
boat	_____	_____
late	_____	_____
feet	_____	_____
We used worms as bait.	_____	_____
He ate the whole pie.	_____	_____
My dad owns a boat.	_____	_____
Why were you late?	_____	_____
My feet are tired.	_____	_____

/d/

Initial Position	Results	Level of Stimulation
do	_____	_____
deck	_____	_____
dog	_____	_____
dime	_____	_____
dam	_____	_____
Do you want to play?	_____	_____
Please sweep the deck.	_____	_____
I have a dog.	_____	_____
It costs a dime.	_____	_____
The dam is big.	_____	_____

Medial Position	Results	Level of Stimulation
ladder	_____	_____
soda	_____	_____
loaded	_____	_____
padded	_____	_____
ready	_____	_____
He climbed the ladder.	_____	_____
I would like a soda.	_____	_____
She loaded up the car.	_____	_____
The chair is padded.	_____	_____
Are you ready yet?	_____	_____

Final Position	Results	Level of Stimulation
bed	_____	_____
fed	_____	_____
head	_____	_____
good	_____	_____
paid	_____	_____
It is time for bed.	_____	_____
Have you fed the cat?	_____	_____
She bumped her head.	_____	_____
This cookie is good.	_____	_____
He got paid yesterday.	_____	_____

/k/

Initial Position	Results	Level of Stimulation
cup	_____	_____
coat	_____	_____
cat	_____	_____
cab	_____	_____
can	_____	_____
Whose cup is this?	_____	_____
I bought a new coat.	_____	_____
I have a nice cat.	_____	_____
Are we taking a cab?	_____	_____
Can you play with me?	_____	_____

Medial Position	Results	Level of Stimulation
bacon	_____	_____
bucket	_____	_____
ticket	_____	_____
jacket	_____	_____
locket	_____	_____
I like to eat bacon.	_____	_____
The bucket is full.	_____	_____
I lost my airline ticket.	_____	_____
Where is your jacket?	_____	_____
I love my locket.	_____	_____

Final Position	Results	Level of Stimulation
ache	_____	_____
take	_____	_____
book	_____	_____
make	_____	_____
sick	_____	_____
I have a bad ache.	_____	_____
Take care of your toys.	_____	_____
I lost my book.	_____	_____
Please make a pie.	_____	_____
Is he sick?	_____	_____

/g/

Initial Position	Results	Level of Stimulation
go	_____	_____
game	_____	_____
gate	_____	_____
goat	_____	_____
gum	_____	_____
May I go outside?	_____	_____
Let's play a game.	_____	_____
Lock the gate.	_____	_____
The goat is fat.	_____	_____
I like to chew gum.	_____	_____

Medial Position	Results	Level of Stimulation
again	_____	_____
soggy	_____	_____
foggy	_____	_____
organ	_____	_____
forget	_____	_____
He is late again.	_____	_____
The bread is soggy.	_____	_____
It is very foggy today.	_____	_____
He can play the organ.	_____	_____
Don't forget the bread.	_____	_____

Final Position	Results	Level of Stimulation
bag	_____	_____
pig	_____	_____
dog	_____	_____
bug	_____	_____
big	_____	_____
Where is my bag?	_____	_____
The pig is pink.	_____	_____
The dog is sick.	_____	_____
He caught a bug.	_____	_____
That is a big bird.	_____	_____

/f/

Initial Position	Results	Level of Stimulation
five	_____	_____
fat	_____	_____
fan	_____	_____
fig	_____	_____
phone	_____	_____
I have five dollars.	_____	_____
That cat is fat.	_____	_____
Please turn on the fan.	_____	_____
I like to eat figs.	_____	_____
He is on the phone.	_____	_____

Medial Position	Results	Level of Stimulation
coffee	_____	_____
safety	_____	_____
waffle	_____	_____
infant	_____	_____
muffin	_____	_____
Do you like coffee?	_____	_____
He ran to safety.	_____	_____
My mom made waffles.	_____	_____
The infant was sick.	_____	_____
The muffin tastes good.	_____	_____

Final Position	Results	Level of Stimulation
half	_____	_____
loaf	_____	_____
beef	_____	_____
cough	_____	_____
cuff	_____	_____
I ate half of my food.	_____	_____
That is a loaf of bread.	_____	_____
Beef comes from cows.	_____	_____
I think I have a cough.	_____	_____
Please cuff your pants.	_____	_____

/v/

Initial Position	Results	Level of Stimulation
vine	_____	_____
vote	_____	_____
vase	_____	_____
van	_____	_____
veil	_____	_____
The long vine is green.	_____	_____
Do not forget to vote.	_____	_____
Put the roses in the vase.	_____	_____
The keys are in the van.	_____	_____
She wore a white veil.	_____	_____

Medial Position	Results	Level of Stimulation
oven	_____	_____
beaver	_____	_____
movie	_____	_____
given	_____	_____
even	_____	_____
Please turn off the oven.	_____	_____
Beavers can swim.	_____	_____
I like the movie.	_____	_____
I was given a chore.	_____	_____
The lines are even.	_____	_____

Final Position	Results	Level of Stimulation
save	_____	_____
leave	_____	_____
shave	_____	_____
wave	_____	_____
dive	_____	_____
Please save me!	_____	_____
Please leave me alone.	_____	_____
My dad needs a shave.	_____	_____
Wave good-bye.	_____	_____
He likes to dive.	_____	_____

/θ/

Initial Position	Results	Level of Stimulation
thin	_____	_____
third	_____	_____
thought	_____	_____
thick	_____	_____
thaw	_____	_____
The line is very thin.	_____	_____
He was third in line.	_____	_____
I thought you left.	_____	_____
This bread is thick.	_____	_____
Thaw out the meat.	_____	_____

Medial Position	Results	Level of Stimulation
author	_____	_____
bathtub	_____	_____
method	_____	_____
toothbrush	_____	_____
Kathy	_____	_____
Who is the author?	_____	_____
The bathtub is clean.	_____	_____
What is your method?	_____	_____
I have a new toothbrush.	_____	_____
Where is Kathy?	_____	_____

Final Position	Results	Level of Stimulation
bath	_____	_____
both	_____	_____
booth	_____	_____
math	_____	_____
path	_____	_____
You need to take a bath.	_____	_____
Are you both going?	_____	_____
He is behind the booth.	_____	_____
I love math.	_____	_____
This is a nice path.	_____	_____

/ð/

Initial Position	Results	Level of Stimulation
the	_____	_____
they	_____	_____
that	_____	_____
this	_____	_____
than	_____	_____
The car is dirty.	_____	_____
They live near you.	_____	_____
That is a big horse.	_____	_____
This is your seat.	_____	_____
Mike is shorter than me.	_____	_____

Medial Position	Results	Level of Stimulation
bother	_____	_____
mother	_____	_____
feather	_____	_____
other	_____	_____
weather	_____	_____
Please don't bother me.	_____	_____
My mother is pretty.	_____	_____
I found a blue feather.	_____	_____
He went the other way.	_____	_____
The weather is bad.	_____	_____

Final Position	Results	Level of Stimulation
clothe	_____	_____
breathe	_____	_____
smooth	_____	_____
bathe	_____	_____
soothe	_____	_____
I will clothe the baby.	_____	_____
Please breathe deeply.	_____	_____
He has smooth skin.	_____	_____
Please bathe tonight.	_____	_____
It will soothe your cut.	_____	_____

/s/

Initial Position	Results	Level of Stimulation
soap	_____	_____
sip	_____	_____
sat	_____	_____
seed	_____	_____
sew	_____	_____
Please wash with soap.	_____	_____
He took a sip of coffee.	_____	_____
Bobby sat on the cake.	_____	_____
I planted the seeds.	_____	_____
Will you sew my dress?	_____	_____

Medial Position	Results	Level of Stimulation
assume	_____	_____
basic	_____	_____
Lassie	_____	_____
lasso	_____	_____
essay	_____	_____
Don't assume anything.	_____	_____
I like basic colors.	_____	_____
Lassie is a smart dog.	_____	_____
He can lasso a horse.	_____	_____
Did you write an essay?	_____	_____

Final Position	Results	Level of Stimulation
face	_____	_____
boss	_____	_____
house	_____	_____
loose	_____	_____
pass	_____	_____
His face is dirty.	_____	_____
My boss is nice.	_____	_____
The house is big.	_____	_____
The dog became loose.	_____	_____
Please pass the salt.	_____	_____

/z/

Initial Position	Results	Level of Stimulation
zip	_____	_____
zoo	_____	_____
zoom	_____	_____
zinc	_____	_____
zero	_____	_____
What is the zip code?	_____	_____
I like to go to the zoo.	_____	_____
The train zoomed by.	_____	_____
The vitamin has zinc.	_____	_____
One minus one is zero.	_____	_____

Medial Position	Results	Level of Stimulation
busy	_____	_____
cousin	_____	_____
diesel	_____	_____
dozen	_____	_____
frozen	_____	_____
She is always busy.	_____	_____
Joe is my cousin.	_____	_____
I have a diesel truck.	_____	_____
We have a dozen cats.	_____	_____
My feet feel frozen.	_____	_____

Final Position	Results	Level of Stimulation
boys	_____	_____
news	_____	_____
has	_____	_____
keys	_____	_____
noise	_____	_____
The boys are playing.	_____	_____
No news is good news.	_____	_____
She has new shoes.	_____	_____
Please hang the keys.	_____	_____
He makes a lot of noise.	_____	_____

/ʃ/

Initial Position	Results	Level of Stimulation
ship	_____	_____
sharp	_____	_____
shop	_____	_____
shake	_____	_____
shoe	_____	_____
The ship set sail.	_____	_____
This pencil is sharp.	_____	_____
I love to shop.	_____	_____
I want a vanilla shake.	_____	_____
Her shoe is dirty.	_____	_____

Medial Position	Results	Level of Stimulation
action	_____	_____
ocean	_____	_____
dishes	_____	_____
bushy	_____	_____
fishing	_____	_____
He likes action movies.	_____	_____
The ocean is blue.	_____	_____
I rinsed the dishes.	_____	_____
Its tail is bushy.	_____	_____
My dad went fishing.	_____	_____

Final Position	Results	Level of Stimulation
fish	_____	_____
wash	_____	_____
push	_____	_____
bush	_____	_____
cash	_____	_____
He likes to fish.	_____	_____
Wash your face.	_____	_____
Don't push your sister.	_____	_____
He hid in the bush.	_____	_____
You must pay cash.	_____	_____

Initial Position	Results	Level of Stimulation
None		

Medial Position	Results	Level of Stimulation
Asia	_____	_____
vision	_____	_____
leisure	_____	_____
treasure	_____	_____
closure	_____	_____
Japan is in Asia.	_____	_____
I have good vision.	_____	_____
She took a leisure trip.	_____	_____
He buried a treasure.	_____	_____
There is a road closure.	_____	_____

Final Position	Results	Level of Stimulation
beige	_____	_____
rouge	_____	_____
massage	_____	_____
collage	_____	_____
mirage	_____	_____
Her pants are beige.	_____	_____
She wears a lot of rouge.	_____	_____
Please massage my neck.	_____	_____
We made a collage.	_____	_____
It was all a mirage.	_____	_____

/h/

Initial Position	Results	Level of Stimulation
hop	_____	_____
he	_____	_____
hat	_____	_____
ham	_____	_____
hot	_____	_____
Rabbits like to hop.	_____	_____
He bought a toy.	_____	_____
She has a nice hat.	_____	_____
I like turkey and ham.	_____	_____
The muffins are hot.	_____	_____

Medial Position	Results	Level of Stimulation
ahead	_____	_____
ahoy	_____	_____
inhale	_____	_____
keyhole	_____	_____
beehive	_____	_____
Please stop ahead.	_____	_____
He shouted, "Ahoy!"	_____	_____
I inhaled the fresh air.	_____	_____
I can't find the keyhole.	_____	_____
Bees live in a beehive.	_____	_____

Final Position	Results	Level of Stimulation
None		

/tʃ/

Initial Position	Results	Level of Stimulation
chair	_____	_____
chip	_____	_____
chess	_____	_____
chap	_____	_____
chin	_____	_____
He sat in the big chair.	_____	_____
I ate lots of chips.	_____	_____
Do you play chess?	_____	_____
The man wore chaps.	_____	_____
Sally hurt her chin.	_____	_____

Medial Position	Results	Level of Stimulation
matches	_____	_____
achieve	_____	_____
catcher	_____	_____
future	_____	_____
inches	_____	_____
Her hair matches mine.	_____	_____
He is a high achiever.	_____	_____
Jerry is the catcher.	_____	_____
We have a bright future.	_____	_____
The line is three inches.	_____	_____

Final Position	Results	Level of Stimulation
beach	_____	_____
peach	_____	_____
catch	_____	_____
itch	_____	_____
rich	_____	_____
I live by the beach.	_____	_____
The peach was sweet.	_____	_____
Catch the ball.	_____	_____
I have a big itch.	_____	_____
My uncle is very rich.	_____	_____

/dʒ/

Initial Position	Results	Level of Stimulation
job	_____	_____
joke	_____	_____
jack	_____	_____
jeep	_____	_____
jaw	_____	_____
Did you take the job?	_____	_____
That was a funny joke.	_____	_____
I read *Jack and Jill*.	_____	_____
I bought a jeep.	_____	_____
Did you hurt your jaw?	_____	_____

Medial Position	Results	Level of Stimulation
digit	_____	_____
cages	_____	_____
digest	_____	_____
agent	_____	_____
magic	_____	_____
This is a two-digit number.	_____	_____
The birds are in cages.	_____	_____
I digested my meal.	_____	_____
He is a secret agent.	_____	_____
I like magic shows.	_____	_____

Final Position	Results	Level of Stimulation
cage	_____	_____
page	_____	_____
stage	_____	_____
edge	_____	_____
huge	_____	_____
The animal is in a cage.	_____	_____
What page are you on?	_____	_____
I danced on the stage.	_____	_____
He sat by the edge.	_____	_____
That is a huge dog.	_____	_____

/w/

Initial Position	Results	Level of Stimulation
wipe	_____	_____
wet	_____	_____
win	_____	_____
wake	_____	_____
we	_____	_____
Wipe your nose.	_____	_____
My clothes are wet.	_____	_____
Did you win the game?	_____	_____
It's time to wake up.	_____	_____
We went on vacation.	_____	_____

Medial Position	Results	Level of Stimulation
away	_____	_____
kiwi	_____	_____
hallway	_____	_____
always	_____	_____
aware	_____	_____
The dog walked away.	_____	_____
Would you like a kiwi?	_____	_____
It's down the hallway.	_____	_____
I always check my work.	_____	_____
Please be aware.	_____	_____

Final Position	Results	Level of Stimulation
None		

/j/

Initial Position	Results	Level of Stimulation
yell	_____	_____
yarn	_____	_____
yolk	_____	_____
yam	_____	_____
use	_____	_____
Don't yell at him.	_____	_____
She knits with yarn.	_____	_____
The egg has a big yolk.	_____	_____
Do you like yams?	_____	_____
Did you use my coat?	_____	_____

Medial Position	Results	Level of Stimulation
royal	_____	_____
kayak	_____	_____
yo-yo	_____	_____
reuse	_____	_____
loyal	_____	_____
The prince is royalty.	_____	_____
I have a red kayak.	_____	_____
Where is my yo-yo?	_____	_____
You can reuse that box.	_____	_____
His friend is loyal.	_____	_____

Final Position	Results	Level of Stimulation
None		

/l/

Initial Position	Results	Level of Stimulation
last	_____	_____
lamb	_____	_____
log	_____	_____
leg	_____	_____
lap	_____	_____
I am always last.	_____	_____
The lamb is lost.	_____	_____
We live in a log cabin.	_____	_____
Is your leg broken?	_____	_____
Can I sit on your lap?	_____	_____

Medial Position	Results	Level of Stimulation
allow	_____	_____
alive	_____	_____
daily	_____	_____
below	_____	_____
chili	_____	_____
He was allowed to go.	_____	_____
The bird is alive.	_____	_____
We get the daily paper.	_____	_____
I hid below the bridge.	_____	_____
I like chili.	_____	_____

Final Position	Results	Level of Stimulation
all	_____	_____
bell	_____	_____
cell	_____	_____
doll	_____	_____
mall	_____	_____
We all ate some cake.	_____	_____
The bell rang loudly.	_____	_____
She has a cell phone.	_____	_____
My doll is lost.	_____	_____
They are at the mall.	_____	_____

/r/

Initial Position	Results	Level of Stimulation
run	_____	_____
rope	_____	_____
rain	_____	_____
rake	_____	_____
rat	_____	_____
Can you run fast?	_____	_____
The rope is long.	_____	_____
It looks like rain.	_____	_____
I like to rake leaves.	_____	_____
I'm afraid of rats.	_____	_____

Medial Position	Results	Level of Stimulation
arrow	_____	_____
carry	_____	_____
fairy	_____	_____
carrot	_____	_____
carol	_____	_____
He shot the arrow.	_____	_____
Will you carry my bag?	_____	_____
I saw a fairy in the yard.	_____	_____
He ate a carrot.	_____	_____
She sang a carol.	_____	_____

Final Position	Results	Level of Stimulation
hair	_____	_____
car	_____	_____
far	_____	_____
door	_____	_____
ear	_____	_____
Her hair is red.	_____	_____
He washed the car.	_____	_____
Do you live far away?	_____	_____
Please lock the door.	_____	_____
My ear hurts.	_____	_____

/m/

Initial Position	Results	Level of Stimulation
mom	_____	_____
mad	_____	_____
mop	_____	_____
man	_____	_____
map	_____	_____
My mom is pretty.	_____	_____
Sue is very mad.	_____	_____
Did you mop the floor?	_____	_____
The man is very nice.	_____	_____
I can't follow a map.	_____	_____

Medial Position	Results	Level of Stimulation
camel	_____	_____
comet	_____	_____
summer	_____	_____
woman	_____	_____
mommy	_____	_____
I saw a camel.	_____	_____
The comet flew by.	_____	_____
Summer is very hot.	_____	_____
That woman is pretty.	_____	_____
I love my mommy.	_____	_____

Final Position	Results	Level of Stimulation
home	_____	_____
ham	_____	_____
game	_____	_____
lime	_____	_____
dim	_____	_____
I want to go home.	_____	_____
Do you like ham?	_____	_____
Let's play a game.	_____	_____
The lime was very sour.	_____	_____
The streetlight is dim.	_____	_____

/n/

Initial Position	Results	Level of Stimulation
no	_____	_____
net	_____	_____
nap	_____	_____
nut	_____	_____
knock	_____	_____
Her father said, "No."	_____	_____
The net is wet.	_____	_____
Let me take a nap.	_____	_____
Do you like nuts?	_____	_____
Please knock first.	_____	_____

Medial Position	Results	Level of Stimulation
bunny	_____	_____
any	_____	_____
many	_____	_____
pony	_____	_____
honey	_____	_____
The bunny is white.	_____	_____
Do you have any pie?	_____	_____
I have many friends.	_____	_____
The pony is small.	_____	_____
Honey is sweet.	_____	_____

Final Position	Results	Level of Stimulation
bean	_____	_____
can	_____	_____
cone	_____	_____
fan	_____	_____
fun	_____	_____
I like bean soup.	_____	_____
Can I go to the zoo?	_____	_____
I want a waffle cone.	_____	_____
Please turn on the fan.	_____	_____
We had a lot of fun.	_____	_____

/ŋ/

Initial Position	Results	Level of Stimulation
None		

Medial Position	Results	Level of Stimulation
hunger	_____	_____
bongo	_____	_____
jungle	_____	_____
singer	_____	_____
finger	_____	_____
He suffers from hunger.	_____	_____
I can play the bongos.	_____	_____
Lions live in the jungle.	_____	_____
She is a singer.	_____	_____
I cut my finger.	_____	_____

Final Position	Results	Level of Stimulation
king	_____	_____
ring	_____	_____
bang	_____	_____
song	_____	_____
wing	_____	_____
John is the king.	_____	_____
He gave her a ring.	_____	_____
I heard a loud bang.	_____	_____
The song was beautiful.	_____	_____
The bird hurt its wing.	_____	_____

PERFORMING A PHONETIC INVENTORY ANALYSIS

A *phonetic inventory analysis* helps the clinician identify the consonants and vowels the child can produce without considering the linguistic contrast of the sound in adult words. In this type of analysis, the clinician is not so much interested in whether the sound was used in the appropriate linguistic or phonetic context, but in whether the child has the **motor** skills to produce the sound. The child's phonetic inventory can be constructed from the information gathered in single-word articulation tests, phonological process assessments, and connected speech samples.

It is important to obtain this information because it gives a broader picture of the child's skills and clinical needs. A phonetic inventory may help the clinician discover that the child can produce only a few sounds or that there is a difference in the child's productive inventory from one word position to another. Furthermore, a phonetic inventory may also show that the child's production of sounds is restricted to certain classes or types of sounds.

Most standardized articulation tests do not include a phonetic inventory analysis form, with the *Khan-Lewis Phonological Assessment, Second Edition* (Khan & Lewis 2002) being an example of one that does. If administering a single-word test that does not include a form for determining a phonetic inventory, the clinician can use **Phonetic Inventory Analysis Form** to supplement assessment data.

Phonetic Inventory Analysis Form

Name: _____

Date of birth: _____

Age: _____

Grade: _____

Teacher: _____

Referred by: _____

Reason for referral: _____

Date: _____

INSTRUCTIONS

- Circle sounds that occur at least three times in each position. These sounds are part of the child's *productive* sound inventory.
- Underline sounds that occur only one or two times in each position. These sounds are *marginal*.

Note

During the assessment, the child did not produce sounds that are neither circled nor underlined, *despite the opportunity to produce them*. These sounds are considered *absent* from the child's phonetic inventory.

Initial Position

m	n	p	b	t	d	k	g	f	v	s	z
θ	ð	ʃ	tʃ	dʒ	w	l	r	j	h		

Medial Position

m	n	ŋ	p	b	t	d	k	g	f	v	s
z	θ	ð	ʃ	ʒ	tʃ	dʒ	w	l	r	j	h

Final Position

m	n	ŋ	p	b	t	d	k	g	f	v	s
z	θ	ð	ʃ	ʒ	tʃ	dʒ	l	r	j		

Vowels and Diphthongs

a	æ	e	ɛ	o	ɔ	u	ʊ	i	ɪ	ə	ʌ
ɚ	ɝ	ai	au	ɔi	ju	eI	ou				

WRITING A DIAGNOSTIC REPORT

Once the assessment has been completed and a diagnosis has been made, the clinician writes a diagnostic report summarizing all of the analyzed information. The diagnostic report provides written documentation of the clinical findings and the treatment recommendations. Because the clinical report becomes an official, and at times legal, document, the clinician should devote sufficient time for its preparation. Also, other professionals often gain some perspective of the clinician's knowledge and competence from the diagnostic report. Reports containing several typographic and grammatical errors, a poor style, and confusing organization and wording may leave a negative impression on the reader.

The exact format, style, length, and degree of detail of clinical reports vary from setting to setting. For example, diagnostic reports written in the university setting are much lengthier and more detailed than those written in other clinical settings. Across settings, diagnostic reports may vary from formatted check-off lists, to one-paragraph reports, to six-page reports. The clinician should be flexible and adhere to the regulations of his or her university program or work setting.

The clinician may use ***Results of Articulation and Phonological Assessment Summary Sheet*** as a general summary of the assessment results and can use the information as an outline for the diagnostic report. ***Sample Diagnostic Reports*** are sample diagnostic reports of articulation and/or phonological disorders.

Results of Articulation and Phonological Assessment Summary Sheet

Name: _____

Date of birth: _____

Age: _____

Grade: _____

Teacher: _____

Referred by: _____

Reason for referral: _____

Teacher Reports

Parent Reports

Birth and Developmental History & Other Pertinent Case History Information

Review of Records

Hearing and Vision Screening Results

Results of Standardized Articulation/Phonological Test

Conversational Speech Sample

Stimulability Testing

Productive Phonetic Inventory

Speech Intelligibility Assessment

Orofacial Examination

Diadochokinetic Syllable Rates

Clinical Impressions and Recommendations

Possible Outside Referrals

_____

Speech–Language Pathologist

Sample Diagnostic Report A: Moderate Articulation Disorder

Oakenshaw Unified School District
Pupil Personnel Services/Special Education
8679 Main Street
Rosevale, CA 95762

INITIAL DIAGNOSTIC REPORT

Name: Cassandra Bennett
School: Jefferson Elementary
Grade: 1
Examiner: Adriana Peña-Brooks,
    M.A., CCC-S

Test date: 10/12/00
Date of birth: 1/8/94
Age: 6-7
Teacher: Mr. Jackson

REFERRAL INFORMATION

Cassandra Bennett, a 6-year-old female, was referred for a speech screening by her classroom teacher, Mr. Jackson, who reported that Cassandra's "s" did not sound correct for her age. After completing a speech screening, this examiner believed that it was appropriate to perform a more thorough evaluation to assess Cassandra's eligibility for speech and language services.

BACKGROUND INFORMATION AND HISTORY

A phone interview was conducted with Mrs. Bennett to obtain relevant developmental information and background history. Mrs. Bennett reported that she was also concerned about Cassandra's "s" production. She indicated that Cassandra has "sounded like this since she started talking."

Cassandra has attended Jefferson Elementary since kindergarten. No prior speech assessments or services were reported. Her developmental history is not remarkable. Mrs. Bennett reported that besides sounding like she always has a cold, Cassandra has enjoyed good health with no significant illnesses.

FAMILY, SOCIAL, AND EDUCATIONAL HISTORY

Cassandra is the first of two children. Mrs. Bennett did not report a family history of communicative disorders. Cassandra attends first grade and is reportedly doing very well in class. She reportedly gets along well with other children. Her classroom teacher characterizes her as "one of the smartest kids in my class." However, he was concerned about the quality of Cassandra's speech.

ASSESSMENT INFORMATION

Cassandra was very cooperative during the testing process. She put forth an appropriate effort with all the tasks presented. Results are thought to present a valid estimate of competency of the skills tested.

Orofacial Examination

An orofacial examination was performed to assess the structure and function of the oral mechanism as related to speech production. Cassandra's lips and hard palate appeared symmetrical at rest. She was able to perform a variety of labial and lingual tasks. The anterior and posterior faucial pillars were within normal limits. Vertical movement of the pharyngeal wall was observed upon the phonation of /a/. Cassandra had enlarged pharyngeal tonsils. A slight overjet also was noted. The bottom central incisors were partially erupted, which created an open space. Cassandra's erupting lower central incisors were discolored. Diadochokinetic syllable rates were within normal limits.

Hearing Screening

The school nurse screened Cassandra's hearing at the beginning of this academic year in August 2000. Results of the screening, as documented in her cumulative folder, were within normal limits. Cassandra passed the hearing screening for the frequencies 250, 500, 1,000, 2,000, and 4,000 at 25 dB HL.

Speech Production and Intelligibility

Cassandra's speech production was assessed with the Photo Articulation Test–3 (PAT–3) and a conversational speech sample. The PAT–3 assesses the production of all English consonants in the initial, medial, and final positions of words according to types of errors (substitutions, omissions, distortions, additions). An analysis of Cassandra's conversational speech sample and her performance on the PAT–3 revealed the following errors:

Target Sound	Initial	Medial	Final
/s/	Dist³/s	Dist³/s	Dist³/s
/z/	Dist³/z	Dist³/z	Dist³/z
/ʃ/	Dist¹/ʃ	Dist¹/ʃ	Dist¹/ʃ
/ʒ/	Dist¹/ʒ	Dist¹/ʒ	Dist¹/ʒ
/dʒ/	Dist¹/dʒ		
/d/	Dist¹/d	Dist¹/d	
/t/	Dist¹/t		

Dist¹ = mild distortion; Dist² = moderate distortion; Dist³ = severe distortion.

Blends

The /s/ component of blends was distorted, as observed in singleton /s/ productions.

Analysis of Cassandra's errors on the speech sample and the PAT–3 revealed that her production of /s/ and /z/ was severely lateralized in all positions of distribution. The consonants /ʃ/, /ʒ/, and /dʒ/ were mildly lateralized. In addition to sibilant distortions, Cassandra demonstrated lateralized production of /d/ in the medial and final positions and distortion of /t/ in the final position of words.

Furthermore, the consonants /ʃ/, /ʒ/, /tʃ/, and /dʒ/ were characterized by the presence of awkward motor movements during their production. While making these sounds, the right side of Cassandra's lower lip deviated down and outward while the upper and lower lips on the left side made contact and became protruded. Although these movements were also noted during production of /tʃ/, the acoustic quality of that sound remained intact.

Cassandra's speech intelligibility was only mildly affected by her misarticulations. A word-by-word analysis of her conversational speech sample revealed that she was 85% intelligible in unknown conversational contexts. Cassandra was highly stimulable for an improved production of /s/ and /z/ in words using modeling and phonetic placement cues. However, other error consonants were not stimulable during this assessment.

Language Production and Comprehension

Cassandra's conversational speech during the assessment showed essentially normal language and structure. Her mean length of utterance was within normal limits for her age. Based on her responses to the examiner's questions and requests, language comprehension appeared adequate.

Voice and Fluency

Cassandra's speech had normal rate and rhythm. The rate of dysfluencies was within the normal range. Therefore, no further analysis of the dysfluency rate was made.

In conversational speech, Cassandra's resonance was perceptually judged to be hyponasal. During a nasal flutter test, her left naris was perceived to be more obstructed than the right. Audible nasal inspiration was also perceived throughout the examination. Mrs. Bennett indicated during a telephone conversation that Cassandra has "sounded like she's had a cold for a very long time."

DIAGNOSTIC SUMMARY AND PROGNOSIS

Cassandra Bennett exhibits a moderate articulation disorder characterized by severe lateralization of /s/ and /z/ and mild lateralization of /ʃ/, /ʒ/, and /ʤ/, /t/, and /d/. Her speech intelligibility was only mildly affected by her articulation errors. Although a slight overjet was noted during the orofacial examination, it is difficult to determine whether this is a contributing factor to her articulation errors. Research has shown that a high percentage of children with slight malocclusions compensate well and have no associated articulation problems.

Cassandra's prognosis for improvement of her misarticulations and her speech intelligibility is good considering her age, adequate language skills, and stimulability for some of the error sounds. Also, Cassandra's parents appear to be very supportive and are anxious to follow through with any home assignments.

RECOMMENDATIONS

Cassandra meets eligibility criteria for language, speech, and hearing services through the school district. Her error productions are atypical in normal development, and she will probably not "outgrow" such sound distortions without clinical intervention. It is recommended that Cassandra receive treatment for her articulation disorder, with an emphasis on improving her production of /s/ and /z/ and other sibilants. It is also recommended that Mrs. Bennett consult with Cassandra's pediatrician regarding her hyponasal quality to rule out any medical problems. Upon Mrs. Bennett's approval, an Individualized Education Program will be developed for Cassandra.

Adriana Peña-Brooks, M.A., CCC-S
Speech–Language Pathologist, License # XXXX

Sample Diagnostic Report B: Severe Phonological Disorder

University Speech and Hearing Clinic
Central University
Central, California 87665

INITIAL DIAGNOSTIC REPORT

Name: Jack Lawson

Address: 1400 General Street

City: Universal, California

Telephone number: (000) 120-5678

Referred by: Mother

Date of birth: 8-2-94

Clinic file number: 00000

Date of report: 9-22-00

Diagnosis: Phonological Disorder

Clinician: Susan Lincoln

BACKGROUND AND PRESENTING COMPLAINT

Jack Lawson, a 6-year-old male, was enrolled in his second semester of speech therapy at the University Clinic on September 15, 2000. Jack's mother served as the informant during this evaluation. The presenting complaint was a severe speech disorder. Mrs. Lawson reported that Jack seems to be "pronouncing words more clearly," is starting to talk more at school, and is using longer sentences. She indicated that she understands approximately 50% of Jack's speech, while others probably understand about 35% when the context of the conversation is known.

HISTORY

Birth, Developmental, and Medical History

Mrs. Lawson reported that her pregnancy was full term and that Jack was born by cesarean section. He weighed 6 pounds, 11 ounces. With the exception of recurrent middle-ear infections, Jack has enjoyed good health with no diseases of significance. Mrs. Lawson reported that Jack had pressure equalization (PE) tubes placed in his ears at approximately 2 years of age. Middle-ear infections were medically treated through antibiotics. According to Mrs. Lawson, a current medical examination revealed that Jack's ears were healthy.

Family, Social, and Educational History

Jack lives with his parents and sister, Karen Lawson. Mrs. Lawson reported that Jack was starting to socialize more with children at school but still tended to play alone. She indicated that Jack does interact with his sister and frequently initiates games to play with her. At the time of this assessment, Jack was attending a day care program at Penter City College. Jack received one semester of speech therapy previously through this clinic. However, there is no other history of speech and language therapy.

OROFACIAL EXAMINATION

An orofacial examination was performed to assess the structural and functional integrity of the oral mechanism. The examination did not reveal anything of clinical significance.

HEARING SCREENING

A bilateral hearing screening was performed at 25 dB HL for 250, 500, 1,000, 2,000, and 4,000 Hz. Jack responded to all frequencies bilaterally.

SPEECH PRODUCTION AND INTELLIGIBILITY

To assess Jack's speech sound production, a conversational speech sample was recorded. In addition, the Goldman-Fristoe Test of Articulation (GFTA) Sounds in Words subtest was administered to assess the production of all English consonants in fixed position. The GFTA assesses the production of sounds according to types of errors (omissions, substitutions, additions, distortions) in initial, medial, and final word positions. An analysis of the sample and Jack's performance on the GFTA revealed the following errors:

Target Sound	Initial	Medial	Final
/k/	t/k	t/k	omit
/g/	d/g	d/g	omit
/ŋ/	nd/ŋ	n/ŋ	
/s/	p/s	t/s	omit
/z/	d/z	d/z	omit
/v/	b/v	b/v	b/v
/ʃ/	t/ʃ	t/ʃ	omit
/ʒ/		d/ʒ	omit
/tʃ/	t/tʃ	t/tʃ	omit
/dʒ/	d/dʒ	d/dʒ	omit
/θ/	f/θ	f/θ	f/θ
/ð/	d/ð	d/ð	d/ð
/r/	w/r	w/r	omit
/l/	w/l	j/l	omit

Blend Errors: k/kl; dw/dr; b/bl; p/pl; fw/fl; kw/kr; tw/sk; t/sl; t/st.
Vowels: No vowel errors were observed.

A phonological process analysis of Jack's speech errors on the Goldman-Fristoe Test of Articulation was performed with the Khan-Lewis Phonological Analysis. The analysis revealed the following phonological processes in the excessive range of usage:

- Deletion of final consonants
- Palatal fronting
- Velar fronting
- Stopping of fricatives and affricates
- Cluster simplification
- Liquid simplification (liquid gliding and vowelization)

Due to the numerous articulation errors and active phonological processes, Jack was found to be 40% intelligible on a word-by-word basis. Jack's speech intelligibility significantly decreased during episodes of a rapid rate of speech and when the length of his utterances increased.

A phonetic inventory analysis revealed the following productive sounds in Jack's speech, according to initial, medial, and final positions:

Initial: [m, n, p, b, t, d, f, w, j, h]
Medial: [m, n, p, b, t, d, f, w, j, h]
Final: [m, n, p, t, d, b]

Stimulability testing revealed limited stimulability for all of the error sounds. Jack made closer approximations of all of the sounds in isolation; however, they did not match the target sound.

LANGUAGE PRODUCTION AND COMPREHENSION

Jack's conversational speech during the assessment showed essentially normal language structure and use except for several missing grammatical morphemes. It is possible that missing grammatical morphemes are due to omission of final consonants. The mean length of utterance (MLU) of his speech sample was 5.7, which is within normal limits for his age.

VOICE AND FLUENCY

Although Jack's speech was difficult to understand, he had normal rate and rhythm. The rate of dysfluencies was within the normal ranges. His voice was also judged to be within normal limits.

DIAGNOSTIC SUMMARY AND PROGNOSIS

Jack Lawson exhibits a severe phonological disorder, which is characterized by several phonological processes, including deletion of final consonants, palatal fronting, velar fronting, stopping of fricatives and affricates, cluster simplification, and liquid simplification (liquid gliding and vowelization). His phonetic inventory was essentially limited to early developing sounds such as stops, nasals, and glides and the fricatives /f/ and /h/. His productive inventory of sounds in the final position of words was limited to [m, n, p, t, d, b], which can help explain the presence of final-consonant deletion. His speech intelligibility was significantly affected by his misarticulations. Jack's phonological disorder may be related to his history of recurrent ear infections during the first 2 years of his life; however, that cannot be conclusively determined to be the cause of his disorder.

Jack is young, was very cooperative during the assessment, and appears to have excellent family support. However, his prognosis for improved phonological skills and speech intelligibility is judged fair at this time due to the severe nature of his disorder, the significant number of articulation errors and phonological processes, and his limited stimulability. His prognosis will be reevaluated throughout the course of therapy.

RECOMMENDATIONS

It is recommended that Jack receive speech–language pathology services, with a focus on increasing his phonetic inventory and decreasing the number of phonological processes. This will likely have a positive effect on his speech intelligibility. As Jack's phonological skills improve, his language may be further evaluated to determine whether morphological features emerge. If they do not, language treatment should be offered.

Submitted by _____
Susan Lincoln, B.A.
Student Clinician

Approved by _____
Adriana Peña-Brooks, M.A., CCC-S
Speech–Language Pathologist
Clinical Supervisor

Parent's Signature _____

Sample Diagnostic Report C: Mild Sound-Specific Articulation Disorder

Mesquite Unified School District
1300 Lancet Avenue
Sunnyvale, California 98675

INITIAL LANGUAGE, SPEECH, AND HEARING EVALUATION

Name: Linda Johnson
School: Palo Verde Elementary
Grade: 3
Examiner: Adriana Peña-Brooks, M.A., CCC-S

Test date: 11/5/02
Date of birth: 11/2/93
Age: 9-0
Teacher: Mrs. Lawson

REFERRAL AND BACKGROUND INFORMATION

Linda Johnson, a third-grade student in Mrs. Lawson's classroom, was referred for a speech screening due to difficulties with "r." After the screening was completed, it was judged that a more thorough assessment was warranted to evaluate her eligibility for articulation services through her public school.

ASSESSMENT RESULTS

Linda was very cooperative throughout testing. She came to the testing room willingly and was friendly and respectful. The results of the assessment were judged to be a valid estimate of her current communication skills.

Linda's voice, fluency, and language skills were judged to be within normal developmental expectations for a student of her age and gender. Testing was limited to an evaluation of her articulation skills using the Photo Articulation Test–3 and a conversational speech sample.

PHOTO ARTICULATION TEST–3 (PAT–3)

The PAT–3 evaluates a student's production of all English consonants in initial, medial, and final position of word according to types of errors (substitutions, omissions, distortions, additions). Linda demonstrated the following consistent errors in all positions of distribution:

- Substitution of w/r
- Significant distortion of syllabic "-er"
- Substitution of /w/ for /r/ component of r-blends

CONVERSATIONAL SPEECH SAMPLE

In conversational speech, Linda consistently substituted w/r and distorted syllabic "-er" as noted during administration of the PAT–3. Linda's speech intelligibility was clinically judged to be 95%–100% in known and unknown contexts.

STIMULABILITY ASSESSMENT

Linda demonstrated poor stimulability for correct production of her error sounds given a model; however, in conversation she was noted to produce "r" correctly in the key word "hundred." She also correctly produced several non-sense words with the "dr" cluster in the medial position (e.g., hundrept, hundrait, hundrick, hundrick, hundrock, and hundrook). She correctly produced the word "Dracula" when coarticulated with the syllable "hun" to produce the word "hunDracula." Linda demonstrated awareness of her difficulties with "r" and "-er" and seemed motivated to improve.

OROFACIAL EXAM

Labial, lingual, and jaw movements were adequate for speech production. Linda had a retainer in place, which she reported she would be wearing for the next year and a half. She was instructed to remove her retainer during testing to obtain a more valid picture of her articulation skills.

SUMMARY AND RECOMMENDATIONS

Linda meets the eligibility criteria for language, speech, and hearing services through the school district for remediation of "r," "-er," and "r-blends," The articulation errors noted are beyond the age of expected development. Although they do not affect her speech intelligibility, they do affect the quality of her speech, and they draw negative attention from her listeners. The results of the testing and recommendations will be shared with her parents and classroom teacher at the scheduled Individualized Education Program (IEP) meeting. Upon approval from Linda's parents, an IEP will be developed to address Linda's current needs.

It has been a pleasure working with Linda. She is a delightful young girl.

Adriana Peña-Brooks, M.A., CCC-S
Speech–Language Pathologist, License SP XXXX

Sample Diagnostic Report D: Profound Phonological Disorder

Greenville Unified School District
121 North Avenue
Eleanor, California 93528

LANGUAGE SPEECH AND HEARING REPORT

Initial Evaluation

Name: JoAnn Stanley
School: Jackson Elementary
Grade: K
Examiner: Adriana Peña-Brooks,
    M.A., CCC-S

Date of report: 9-26-00
Date of birth: 5-01-95
Age: 5-4
Teacher: Mrs. Thomas

REFERRAL INFORMATION

JoAnn Stanley, a 5-year-old female, was referred for a speech screening by her classroom teacher, Mrs. Thomas. According to Mrs. Thomas, JoAnn's "placement of sounds in words is mixed up." After completing a general screening, this examiner believed that a more thorough assessment was warranted to determine JoAnn's eligibility for speech and language services through an Individualized Education Program (IEP).

BACKGROUND INFORMATION AND HISTORY

A phone interview was conducted with Mrs. Stanley and a child case history form was sent home to obtain information on JoAnn's developmental history. Mrs. Stanley completed the case history form and reported that JoAnn is one of three children. She has an older sister, Megan, and a younger brother, Eli. Her mother works inside the home, and her father is a computer programmer.

Mrs. Stanley reported that JoAnn "communicates in sentences but has really bad babytalk and also talks with her teeth clenched." She has a history of fluid buildup behind her ears that, according to Mrs. Stanley, went undetected until she was 4 years old. She has had three ear infections since birth and had an adenoidectomy at age 4. Mrs. Stanley believed that the removal of JoAnn's adenoids helped the quality of her speech. A full audiological evaluation after her adenoidectomy showed her hearing to be within normal limits.

Mrs. Stanley reported that JoAnn's communication and motor skills developed as expected with the exception of her articulation skills.

ASSESSMENT INFORMATION AND TEST RESULTS

JoAnn was very cooperative during the testing process. Results were judged to be an accurate estimate of her communication skills.

SPEECH PRODUCTION AND INTELLIGIBILITY

JoAnn's articulation-phonological skills were assessed with the Test of Minimal Articulation Competence (T-MAC) and a conversational speech sample. The T-MAC assesses the production of all English consonants in prevocalic, intervocalic, and postvocalic positions. It also assesses several vowels, diphthongs, and blends. The following results were obtained:

Target Sound	Prevocalic	Intervocalic	Postvocalic
p	+	?/p	omit/p
b	+	+	omit/b
t	+	+	omit/t
d	+	+	omit/d
k	+	?/k	omit/k
g	+	d/g	omit/g
s	+	?/s	omit/s
z	s/z	/z	omit/z
ʃ	+	?/ʃ	?/ʃ
ʒ	----	?/ʒ	omit/ʒ
θ	f/θ	h/θ	omit/θ
ð	+	d/ð	omit ð
f	+	s/f	omit/f
v	f/v	b/v	b/v
h	+	+	----
ʧ	+	?/ʧ	omit/
ʤ	+	+	omit/ʤ
m	+	+	+
n	+	+	+
ŋ	----	n/ŋ	omit/ŋ

w	+	+	----
j	+	+	----
l	+	+	omit/l
r	w/r	w/r	----

Note: The "----" mark indicates that the sound was either not tested or does not occur in that position. The "+" mark indicates the sound was produced correctly.

Blends: p/sp, t/st, s/sn, k/sk, s/sm, pw/pr, bw/br, fw/fr, fw/thr, tw/tr, dw/dr, gw/gr, kw/kr.

Vowels: JoAnn correctly produced all vowels tested with exception of /ɝ/ and the centering diphthongs / Iɚ, ɛɚ, ɑɚ, and ɔɚ/.

When JoAnn's errors were analyzed according to phonological processes, the following significant (20% + percentage of occurrence) patterns were identified: final consonant deletion, replacement of a glottal stop for medial plosives, syllable deletion, inconsistent velar fronting, stopping, cluster reduction, liquid gliding, and vowelization.

A conversational speech sample revealed essentially the same error patterns identified during administration of the T-MAC. Her speech intelligibility was clinically judged to be 30%–40% in unknown contexts and approximately 50% in known and highly structured contexts. A child of her chronological age would be expected to be approximately 90% intelligible in known and unknown contexts. JoAnn was highly stimulable for correct production of the error sounds and phonological patterns.

OROFACIAL EXAMINATION

An orofacial examination was performed to rule out an organic, structural, or neurological variable as the underlying cause of JoAnn's articulation-phonological errors. Nothing of clinical significance was noted, with exception of a slight overbite. Mrs. Stanley reported that JoAnn underwent extensive dental work at the age of 2. During the orofacial examination, it was noted that several of her lower molars were capped and her four upper front teeth were crowned.

LANGUAGE

JoAnn's receptive and expressive language skills were judged to be within normal limits for her chronological age based on informal observations. However, her syntactic and morphologic development should be closely monitored as her speech intelligibility increases because many morphological markers are produced by final consonants, and JoAnn currently omits most final consonants. The Peabody Picture Vocabulary Test-III was administered to obtain a general indication of JoAnn's receptive vocabulary for pictured words. She received a standard score of 95, which falls within the average range.

DIAGNOSTIC STATEMENT

Results of the T-MAC and a conversational speech sample revealed a profound phonological disorder. She displayed many substitution errors that, when analyzed according to phonological processes, were identified as final consonant deletion, replacement of a glottal stop for medial plosives, syllable deletion, inconsistent velar fronting, stopping, cluster reduction, liquid gliding, and vowelization. JoAnn was highly stimulable for correct production of the target sounds and phonological patterns.

SUMMARY AND RECOMMENDATIONS

JoAnn meets the eligibility criteria for speech and language services for articulation and phonological therapy. The articulation-phonological errors observed during testing profoundly affect her speech intelligibility. If left untreated, JoAnn's phonological disorder will very likely affect her social and academic interactions. Therefore, speech and language services are highly recommended through an Individualized Education Program. The results of testing will be shared with JoAnn's parents and classroom teacher during the scheduled IEP qualifying meeting, and a team decision regarding the most appropriate educational program for JoAnn will be made at that time.

It was a pleasure working with JoAnn. She is a friendly and pleasant young girl. Please feel free to contact me at _____ if you have any questions or concerns.

_____

Adriana Peña-Brooks, M.A., CCC-S
Speech–Language Pathologist, License # XXXX

Sample Diagnostic Report E: Articulation and Language Disorder

General Unified School District
121 E. Lakefront Street
Grand Lake, California 83678

INITIAL LANGUAGE, SPEECH, AND HEARING REPORT

Name: John Lancet
School: Successful Elementary
Grade: 1
Examiner: Adriana Peña-Brooks,
M.A., CCC-S

Date of report: 04-04-2001
Date of birth: 10-02-93
Age: 7-5
Teacher: Mrs. Stockton

REFERRAL INFORMATION

John Lancet, a 7-year-old first-grade student, was referred for a speech and language screening by his classroom teacher, who expressed concerns about his speech articulation, speech fluency, and vocal quality ("nasal quality, too soft"). The speech and language screening was completed on February 15, 2001, and at that time oral-motor weaknesses, articulation delays, and other speech issues were identified as areas that warranted further examination. The results of the screening were shared with John's mother over the telephone.

The school resource specialist screened John's reading skills and in the process identified some difficulties with his oral reading fluency. A Student Study Team (SST) meeting was held on February 26, 2001, to address John's speech and academic needs. The team decided that John would benefit from a full speech and language examination to determine his eligibility for services under an Individualized Education Program (IEP). The team also recommended informal support in the Learning Center for improvement of his oral reading fluency. Mr. and Mrs. Lancet agreed to the speech and language assessment on the day of the SST meeting and signed appropriate paperwork. They also agreed that John should receive informal academic support in the Learning Center.

BACKGROUND AND HISTORY INFORMATION

A child case history form was sent home to John's parents for completion to gain a better understanding of his family and developmental history. Mrs. Lancet completed the case history form. John is one of seven children. He has two older brothers, Robert and Steven, an older sister, Brianna, and three younger brothers, Bill, Thomas, and Greg. His mother, Mrs. Rose Lancet, works inside the home and his father, Mr. Michael Lancet, is a warehouse supervisor.

Mrs. Lancet indicated in the case history form that John has difficulty "forming complete sentences and some letter sounds." She further reported that John usually communicates in single words, gestures, and short phrases. She first noticed the problem "a couple of years ago with certain words. Mrs. Stockton and Mrs. Pena-Brooks noticed it this year." She attributed the problem to a tongue thrust, which was identified by his dentist a few weeks ago. Mrs. Lancet indicated that John's speech and language has slightly improved from a couple of years ago when she first noticed the problem. She further indicated that John does not seem to be aware of the problem.

Mrs. Lancet indicated that her general health during her pregnancy with John was good. Her pregnancy was full term and he weighed 8 pounds at birth. All developmental milestones were reported to be within normal limits. Mrs. Lancet did indicate that although John does not have difficulty walking or running, he is not very coordinated. His classroom teacher reported that John tends to trip and stumble over things in class. John's mother described him as a child who "is shy at first, but very friendly, loving, and playful."

At the recommendation of this examiner, Mrs. Lancet took John to a doctor to rule out any medical problems that could be related to the oral motor weaknesses identified during the speech screening and the poor motor coordination observed at home and in the classroom. Mrs. Lancet indicated that John "met with his doctor in February of 2001. She felt he was okay. He was a little slow with some motor exercises. His hearing and vision were both fine." John passed a vision and hearing screening completed by the school nurse at Successful Elementary on April 4, 2001.

ASSESSMENT RESULTS

John was very cooperative during the testing process. Results were judged to be an accurate estimate of the skills tested.

SPEECH

Test of Minimal Articulation Competence (T-MAC)

John's articulation skills were assessed with the *Test of Minimal Articulation Competence* (T-MAC) and a spontaneous speech sample. The T-MAC assesses the production of all English consonants in prevocalic, intervocalic, and postvocalic positions. It also assesses several vowels, diphthongs, and blends.

The following substitution errors were observed: f/θ in final position and θ/f in final position. John's production of all other consonants, blends, vowels, and diphthongs were correct according to place of production, meaning that they were made where expected along the oral cavity. However, the majority of his consonants, stop-plosives, fricatives, and affricates in particular, were imprecise. They were generally too soft, weak in production, and lacked adequate intraoral pressure. He was not stimulable for improved production of stop-plosives, fricatives, and affricates when given an exaggerated model.

Speech Sample

A conversational speech sample revealed the same consonant error patterns identified during administration of the T-MAC. It was noted that his breathing pattern was affected, in that he needed to take a new breath every few words (three to four words). Most of his air supply was used up on the first few words forcing him to speak on residual air for the latter part of his utterance. This resulted in sound and syllable omissions in his connected words. His resonance quality was hyponasal. He showed very little inflectional and volume changes in his utterances, resulting in a monotone and monoloud quality. Considering all of the patterns identified, his speech was judged to have a dysarthric quality. His speech intelligibility was clinically judged to be 40% in unknown contexts and approximately 50% in known and highly structured contexts. A child of his chronological age would be expected to be nearly 90% intelligible in known and unknown contexts.

Orofacial Examination

An orofacial examination was performed to assess the structure and function of the speech mechanism. Visual inspection of the oral cavity revealed a high, narrow palate. Structure of the soft palate appeared normal; however, slow and limited backward and upward movement was observed during production of "ah." The structure of the tongue and the lips were within normal limits. However, when asked to extend, elevate, and lateralize his tongue and stretch and purse his lips, John's movements were generally slow and had limited range of movement. When asked to open and close his jaw several times continuously, his movements were very slow. Diadochokinetic syllables rates were below age-level expectations. His production of "pu-pu-pu," "tu-tu-tu," "ku-ku-ku," and "pu-tu-ku" were slow and labored, and articulation was imprecise. A significant overbite was noted upon visual inspection. According to Mrs. Lancet, John's dentist indicated that his overbite was related to a tongue thrust pattern. A mouth-breathing pattern was observed.

LANGUAGE

Peabody Picture Vocabulary Test–IIIA (PPVT–IIIA)

The PPVT–IIIA is a receptive vocabulary measure. The student is asked to point to a black and white picture representing a word spoken by the examiner (e.g., "Point to the locket") from a choice of four. The words start simple and become more difficult as the test progresses. John obtained the following results:

Raw Score = 96

Standard Score = 98

Percentile Rank = 45

Age Equivalent = 7-2

Description: Average skills

Standard Score Mean = 100; Standard Deviation = 15; scores between 85 to 115 are in the average range.

Expressive One-Word Picture Vocabulary Test (EOWPVT)

The EOWPVT is an expressive single-word vocabulary measure. The student is asked to verbally label a white and black drawing representing a word (e.g., "What is this?"). John's scores were as follows:

Raw Score = 77

Standard Score = 107

Percentile Rank = 68

Age Equivalent = 8–4

Description: Average skills

Standard Score Mean = 100; Standard Deviation = 15; scores between 85 to 115 are in the average range.

John's performance on the PPVT III–A and EOWPVT was in the average range. He seems to have acquired a solid foundation in his receptive and expressive vocabulary skills for adequate understanding and expression of important terms and concepts introduced and discussed in the classroom setting.

Clinical Evaluation of Language Fundamentals–Revised (CELF–R)

The CELF–R was administered to assess John's receptive and expressive language skills. This test assesses a variety of receptive and expressive syntactic, semantic, and morphologic language skills. John's performance on this assessment instrument was as follows:

	Raw Score	Standard Score	%ile Rank
		Receptive Language Subtests	
• Linguistic Concepts	17	9	37
• Sentence Structure	25	12	75
• Oral Directions	6	5	5
Receptive Language Score		**91**	**27**
		Expressive Language Subtests	
• Word Structure	31	9	37
• Formulated Sentences	32	6	9
• Recalling Sentences	46	8	25
Expressive Language Score		**84**	**14**
Total Language Score		**86**	**18**
		Supplementary Subtests	
• Listening to Paragraphs	7	10	50

John's performance on the CELF–R revealed low-average receptive language skills, although a significant weakness was noted in the following oral directions subtest. He had particular difficulties following two- and three-step oral directions. His expressive language skills were in the borderline range of performance, with the most notable area of weakness being in formulating sentences when given a key word. Some of John's sentences were incomplete phrases. His Total Langue Score (Receptive and Expressive scores combined) was in the low-average range.

LANGUAGE SAMPLE

During a spontaneous sample collected in the speech room, John tended to use single words and simple phrases. His verbal output was limited for a child of his chronological age. His mother provided this examiner with a home language sample. John's sentences were somewhat longer, averaging five to six words. Morphological and syntactic structures in his sentences were within normal developmental limits.

SUMMARY AND RECOMMENDATIONS

John meets the eligibility criteria for DIS-LSH services due to moderate articulation, speech, and oral-motor delays that affect the quality and intelligibility of his speech. Weaknesses were also noted in his ability to follow two- and three-step oral directions and his ability to formulate sentences on demand. John's moderate speech and language delays are likely to impinge on his academic performance (e.g., following directions in the classroom, understanding teacher directions, reading fluency, oral presentations, generating verbal and written sentences on demand, and so forth). Speech and language services are highly recommended to help John overcome some of his current weaknesses. Results of testing will be shared with John's parents and classroom teacher during the scheduled IEP team meeting. Upon approval by his parents, an Individualized Education Program will be developed to meet John's current individual needs.

It was a pleasure working with John. He is a cooperative and pleasant young boy. I look forward to working with John in the future.

_____

Adriana Peña-Brooks, M.A., CCC-S
Speech–Language Pathologist, License # XXXX

Sample Diagnostic Report F: Articulation and Language Disorder Related to Hearing Loss

Sierra Desert Unified School District
86790 Montana Avenue
Rancho Agua Azul, California 98678

LANGUAGE, SPEECH, AND HEARING REPORT: TRIENNIAL REEVALUATION

Name: Skyler Tamaki
School: Sierra Elementary
Grade: 1
Teacher: Mrs. Lopez

Tests dates: 3-15-02 & 3-22-02
Date of birth: 10-4-95
Age: 6-5
Examiner: Adriana Peña-Brooks, M.A., CCC-S

REFERRAL AND BACKGROUND INFORMATION

Skyler Tamaki, a 6-year-old first grader, was initially evaluated in April of 1999 by Linda Peters, a speech-language pathologist with the Early Intervention Program/Phonological Clinic at Montana Elementary. He was diagnosed with a severe phonological process disorder that significantly affected his speech intelligibility. Initial testing also revealed significant delays in his oral grammar (syntax and morphology) skills. Skyler was subsequently diagnosed with bilateral high-frequency sensorineural hearing loss in October of 1999, and behind-the-ear hearing aids were placed in both ears. He received group therapy at the Phonological Clinic during the 1998-1999 and 1999-2000 school years. He entered kindergarten at Sierra Elementary in July of 2000 with an active Individualized Education Program (IEP) for articulation and oral grammar therapy, at which time he started receiving speech therapy services two times a week, 30 minutes per session in a small group setting.

Skyler currently wears Unitron FX (taupe) hearing aids in both ears. According to Mrs. Tamaki, a recent audiological evaluation revealed no further loss in hearing from his previous exam on January 31, 2001. Mrs. Tamaki reported that Skyler will receive new hearing aids in November of 2002.

This report is part of Skyler's triennial reevaluation, which is required by federal regulations to evaluate his progress over the last 3 years and to determine his continued need for services.

TEST RESULTS AND INTERPRETATION

Skyler put forth an appropriate effort with the tasks presented. He was generally cooperative and attentive to task despite his physical activity. As observed in therapy, he is a very active boy who benefits from high structure and clear expectations. Results of testing are thought to present a valid estimate of his current communication skills.

SPEECH

Test of Minimal Articulation Competence (T-MAC)

The *Test of Minimal Articulation Competence* was given to Skyler on March 22, 2002, to obtain a current assessment of his articulation skills at the fixed-position word level. The T-MAC assesses English consonants in prevocalic, intervocalic, and postvocalic positions. It also assesses the production of some blends, the majority of vowels, and some diphthongs. Skyler produced the following errors:

Target	Prevocalic	Intervocalic	Postvocalic
/t/	correct	correct	unreleased
/s/	distorted	distorted	θ/z
/z/	correct	correct	distorted /s/
/ʒ/		ʤ/ʒ	ʤ/ʒ
/θ/	correct	correct	distorted /θ/
/l/	correct	correct	omit/l

Blends: p/sp, t/st, θl/sl, tk/sk, tw/sw, m/sm, l/sl, bw/bl, pw/pl, k/kl
Vowels and Diphthongs: All vowels and diphthongs were produced correctly.

LANGUAGE

Peabody Picture Vocabulary Test-IIIA (PPVT-IIIA)

The PPVT-IIIA was administered to assess Skyler's listening vocabulary development. During this test, the student is asked to point to a black and white picture representing a word spoken by the examiner (e.g., "Point to locket") from a choice of four items. The words start simple and become progressively more difficult. Skyler obtained the following results:

Raw Score = 86

Standard Sore = 100

Percentile Rank = 50

Age Equivalent = 6-6

Description: Average skills

Skyler's performance on the PPVT–IIIA revealed age-appropriate receptive vocabulary. He appears to be acquiring vocabulary as expected for a child of his age despite his moderate-severe hearing loss.

CONVERSATIONAL SPEECH AND LANGUAGE

Skyler is an extremely verbal boy who enjoys social interactions. He expresses his thoughts and ideas in a logical and sequenced manner. His mean length of utterance is adequate for his age, although he continues to make occasional morphosyntactic (grammatical) errors, particularly with subject-verb agreement, plurality, and past-tense markers. He continues to make inconsistent articulation errors of "s" and "z" during natural conversational interactions. When produced in error, his "s" and "z" productions continue to be interdentalized or stopped. He also misarticulates /l/ and /θ/ inconsistently. His "s" and "l" blends are affected by his misarticulations of singleton /s/ and /l/. His speech intelligibility was judged to be at least 95% during natural conversational interactions despite the presence of some articulation errors.

OROFACIAL EXAMINATION

As documented in past reports, Skyler's structure and function of the lips, tongue, and jaw are within normal limits. Nothing of clinical significance was noted during his most current orofacial examination.

THERAPY OBSERVATIONS

In therapy sessions, Skyler can produce "s" and "z" with at least 90% accuracy in words and simple sentences with high structure. His production of "s" and "z" improves in its strident quality when he uses a "tongue-tip up" versus a "tongue-tip down" position. His accuracy decreases in natural conversational interactions where it has not been specified that his productions will be monitored and charted. He occasionally misarticulates "l," particularly when it occurs in consonant blends. Skyler's self-monitoring skills have been slow to develop.

SUMMARY AND RECOMMENDATIONS

Skyler has made very good progress in his articulation and language skills over the last 3 years. The severity of his articulation disorder has improved from severe to mild-moderate. However, he continues to produce distortions of "s" and "z" and occasional misarticulations of "l" in natural conversational interactions. He also continues to demonstrate mild difficulties in his oral grammar skills. His articulation and grammar weaknesses are likely related to his moderate-severe sensorineural hearing loss. Therefore, it is strongly recommended that he continue to receive speech and language services to address his continued areas of need. The results of the assessment will be reviewed at the scheduled IEP meeting where his continued eligibility for services will be determined.

It has been a pleasure working with Skyler. He is a vivacious and charming young man with a funny and warm personality. I wish him great success in the future.

Adriana Peña-Brooks, M.A., CCC-S
Speech–Language Pathologist, License # XXXX

Part III
Treatment Resources

CHOOSING POTENTIAL GOALS AND OBJECTIVES

After completing an assessment of a child's articulation and phonological skills, the clinician identifies the potential treatment goals and objectives. *Short-term objectives* refer to skills that can be trained in a relatively short period of time (e.g., two weeks, one month, three months). They are steps toward achieving the long-term goal. *Long-term goals* are the articulation or phonological skills that the child is expected to learn by the end of a specified treatment period (e.g., one semester in most university settings and one year in most public school settings). Adequate long-term goals and short-term objectives can be established only if the child is seen as an individual and his or her special needs are carefully considered.

General Principles for the Selection of Target Behaviors and *Clinical Guidelines on Target Behavior Selection* outline general principles to be considered in the selection of articulation and phonological targets treatment. See the "Basic Unit" of Chapter 8 in *Assessment and Treatment of Articulation and Phonological Disorders* for an in-depth review of the selection of target behaviors.

CONSIDERATIONS FOR SELECTING INDIVIDUAL SOUNDS

- Select target sounds that are part of the child's phonetic repertoire (as determined by a phonetic inventory analysis). Alternatively, select those that are not part of the child's phonetic inventory; preferably, select some that are part of the child's phonetic inventory and some that are not and see which methods work the best.
- Select target sounds for which the child is most stimulable. Alternatively, select those that are not stimulable; preferably, select some that are stimulable and some that are not and see which approach works the best.
- Select target sounds the child inconsistently misarticulates; alternatively, select only those that are consistently misarticulated.
- Select target sounds that have the highest potential to increase speech intelligibility.
- Select target sounds that are frequently occurring.
- Select target sounds that develop early; alternatively, select sounds that are late developing to see which strategy works the best.
- Select target sounds that the child or family most desires to correct.
- Select target sounds that are more visible and potentially easier for the child to learn; alternatively, select sounds that are difficult to see to identify which strategy works the best.

CONSIDERATIONS FOR SELECTING PHONOLOGICAL PROCESSES

- Select processes that are inconsistent or unstable—in other words, those that have a low frequency of occurrence (processes that are on their way out); alternatively, select processes that have a high frequency of occurrence and see which methods work the best for an individual child.
- Select processes that occur only in certain phonetic environments; alternatively, select processes that occur consistently across phonetic environments to see which strategy works the best.
- Select processes that affect sounds that are within the child's phonetic inventory. These are sounds that the child can produce to some extent, though not always in the appropriate linguistic context to create a contrast between words; alternatively, select processes that affect sounds that are not yet within the child's phonetic inventory and see which strategy works the best.
- Select processes that affect sounds for which the child is stimulable. Alternatively, select processes that affect sounds that are not stimulable to see which strategy works the best.
- Select processes that are deviant, unusual, or idiosyncratic. For example, velarization, lateralization, frication of stops, and glottal replacement may make good initial targets

since they may call more attention to the child's speech than more common processes such as cluster reduction.

- Select processes that contribute significantly to the child's reduced intelligibility. Stopping, for example, may have a significant effect on the child's speech intelligibility since it can affect a large set of sounds.
- Select processes that result in extensive homonymy. Homonymy leads to the loss of linguistic contrast between two or more words (e.g., child produces [pɪt] for "his," "fish," and "sit" due to the effects of stopping of fricatives) and may significantly affect speech intelligibility.
- Select "early" processes or processes that affect early sounds; alternatively, select processes that affect later-developing sounds and see which approach works best for a particular child.

Clinical Guidelines on Target Behavior Selection

If the goal of therapy is the child's immediate success over other factors such as generalized productions and marked improvement on speech intelligibility, then consider

- sounds that are easier to teach;
- sounds that are stimulable;
- sounds that are produced with better than zero frequency on baseline trials;
- sounds that are visible;
- sounds that are in any way easier for a given child because of individual differences (e.g., child may find it easier to learn an intuitively complex sound than a simple sound);
- individual sound errors that are inconsistent (i.e., produced correctly in some contexts);
- phonological processes that occur significantly below 100% (i.e., processes that are on their way out).

If the goal of therapy is to choose targets that may lead to immediate generalized productions and markedly improved speech intelligibility, select as treatment targets

- sounds that are complex;
- sounds that are consistently misarticulated;
- sounds that are nonexistent in the child's phonetic repertoire;
- phonological processes that affect the greatest number of sounds;
- phonological processes that are idiosyncratic or unusual;
- phonological processes that reduce *homonymy*;
- phonological processes that are exhibited in 100% of opportunities or close to it.

Regardless of initial success or generalization considerations, select as treatment targets

- sounds that are ethnoculturally appropriate for the child;
- sounds that are in the child's dialect;
- sounds that are not in the dialect only if the child or family demand their treatment;
- sounds in words that are important in view of the child's academic success (i.e., reading assignments, language work in the classroom, literacy considerations);
- sounds in words that are most frequently used in the child's language;
- sounds that are still produced in error or phonological processes that are still active regardless of previous guidelines followed.

ESTABLISHING BASELINES

Assessment data, though essential in making a diagnosis, may not be adequate for establishing a reliable and valid pretreatment performance measure that will help evaluate the child's progress over time. Many traditional standardized articulation tests allow minimal opportunities—often only three—for the occurrence of a specific speech sound or phonological process. If the child misarticulates the sound during administration of the articulation test, it may be incorrectly assumed that he or she has not mastered production of the sound. Also, test results do not help calculate the accuracy percentage with which the child produces various sounds. Baselines overcome these limitations.

Baselines are measured rates of behaviors in the absence of treatment. They provide detailed pretreatment information that can be used to (a) evaluate the child's progress over time, (b) establish treatment effectiveness (or ineffectiveness), and (c) establish clinician accountability. The clinician follows four general steps to establish baselines of potential target behaviors: (1) *specify the treatment targets in measurable terms*, (2) *prepare the stimulus items*, (3) *prepare a recording sheet*, and (4) *administer the baseline trials*.

Baseline Recording Sheet is a data sheet that the clinician can use to record the client's baseline performance; it can be modified to meet the individual child's needs. See the "Basic Unit" of Chapter 8 in *Assessment and Treatment of Articulation and Phonological Disorders* for more information on baseline procedures.

Baseline Recording Sheet

Name: _____ Age: _____ Clinician: _____

Date: _____ Disorder(s) : _____

Potential Target Behavior: _____

(+) = correct   (−) = incorrect   (NR) = no response

Target Response	Evoked Trials +/−/ NR	Modeled Trials +/−/ NR	Prompted Trials +/−/ NR
1.			
2.			
3.			
4.			
5.			
6.			
7.			
8.			
9.			
10.			
11.			
12.			
13.			
14.			
15.			
16.			
17.			
18.			
19.			
20.			
Percentage Correct			

DEVELOPING MEASURABLE GOALS AND OBJECTIVES

After identifying potential target behaviors, the clinician defines the target behaviors in measurable terms. The components of a measurable target can vary depending on the child's skills and treatment needs, and the style in which they are written may need to be suited to a specific clinical setting. The quality of the statement should not suffer by such variations. By asking the following questions, the clinician can ensure that the important components of a measurable objective are included:

- *Did I state the skill I want the child to learn or perform?* (Response topography)
- *Did I indicate the accuracy criterion or performance level I expect the child to reach?* (A quantitative criterion)
- *Did I indicate the mode in which I want the child to respond?* (Response mode)
- *Did I indicate at what linguistic level I expect the child to use the new skill?* (Response level)
- *Did I indicate under what circumstances or situations I expect the child to use the taught skills?* (Number of speech samples or sessions)

The clinician may refer to **Sample Treatment Goals and Objectives** for examples of measurable treatment objectives for articulation and phonological disorders.

The following is a sampling of measurable short-term objectives for individual sounds, phonological processes, distinctive features, and other behaviors that may contribute to improved articulation and phonological skills. The clinician may alter the sample goals to fit the needs of the individual child.

TREATMENT OBJECTIVES FOR INDIVIDUAL SOUNDS

- A minimum of 90% correct evoked production of /s/ and /z/ in single words across three clinical sessions.
- At least 90% correct production of /f/ in conversational speech produced at the clinic, at school, and in the child's home across three speech samples.
- Production of initial /d/ with 80% accuracy in 10 untrained words during evoked trials in the clinical setting.
- Spontaneous production of /k/ and /g/ in sentences with 90% accuracy over three consecutive sessions in response to the clinician's questions.
- Correct production of /s/ in the initial position or words used in two-word phrases evoked on a set of 20 discrete trials at 90% accuracy.

TREATMENT OBJECTIVES FOR PHONOLOGICAL PROCESSES

- The reduction of final consonant deletion by teaching 90% correct production of the following sounds in the word-final position measured across three clinical sessions: /p/, /k/, /t/, and /m/.
- The elimination of stopping by teaching 90% correct production of the following fricatives at the conversational level measured in three treatment sessions: /s/, /f/, /θ/, and /ʃ/.
- The reduction of syllable deletion by training 20 client-specific multisyllabic words in two-word phrases with 90% accuracy observed across three sessions.
- To eliminate the presence of velar fronting by training 90% correct production of /k/, /g/, and /ŋ/ in conversational speech across three speech samples gathered in the client's home.
- To establish the contrast between singleton consonants and consonant clusters by training 80% correct production of the following /s/ + stop clusters in the initial position of words: /st/, /sp/, and /sk/.

TREATMENT OBJECTIVES FOR DISTINCTIVE FEATURES

- To establish the nasality feature by training 90% correct production of the following exemplars in words while naming pictured objects in three consecutive clinical sessions: /m/ and /n/.

- To establish the [+ voice/-voice] feature contrast by training 90% correct production of the following cognate pairs in two-word phrases measured across three consecutive treatment sessions: [p-b], [k-g], [f-v], and [s-z].
- To establish the stridency feature by training at least 90% correct production of /s/, /ʃ/, and /ʧ/ in evoked word trials across three consecutive treatment sessions. Generalized production of the stridency feature to the untrained cognate pairs will be probed when the client reaches the initial training criterion.
- To establish the [continuant-interrupted] feature contrast by training 90% correct production of the following sound exemplars of the [+ continuant] feature in single words: /f/, /s/, and /ʃ/ measured across three consecutive treatment sessions. Minimal pairs (e.g., *pan-fan, two-shoe,* and *top-shop*) will be incorporated for contrast training, and generalized productions to the untrained cognate pairs will be assessed.

OTHER POSSIBLE TREATMENT OBJECTIVES

- To eliminate the presence of *homonymous word forms* by training 90% correct production or acceptable approximation of the following words in three consecutive sessions: (*list words affected by homonymy*).
- To increase the client's phonetic repertoire of sound by training 90% correct production of the following consonants: /t/, /k/, /s/, and /f/. The client will be expected to produce each sound in a set of 10 untrained words at the sentence level during evoked discrete trials.
- To train a reduced rate of speech to facilitate precise articulatory contacts in conversational speech. The client will be expected to maintain a rate of 125 words per minute across three 10-minute conversational speech samples in the home situation.
- To increase the client's use of varying **syllable word shapes** by targeting at least 80% correct production of [C-V-C], [CCVC], and [CVCC] words in sentences in three consecutive clinical sessions.
- At least 90% accuracy in self-correcting articulation errors of /s/ and /z/ in conversational speech observed across three consecutive treatment sessions.

> *These objectives are not meant to be exhaustive, and they should be tailored to the individual child's needs. The response mode, response level, accuracy criterion, and stimulus conditions should be altered to fit the child's assessment and baseline performance. The clinician's own treatment philosophy and the child's specific diagnosis often dictate whether the target behaviors will be written in terms of individual phonemes, phonological processes, distinctive features, or a combination of these.*

COLLECTING TREATMENT DATA

It is imperative that the clinician collect the child's performance data in treatment to (a) quantify the child's progress, (b) evaluate the effectiveness of treatment, and (c) establish professional accountability. All employment settings require some level of documentation of the child's progress, so it is important that the clinician devise or adapt recording forms that permit such documentation. In articulation therapy, the clinician can judge the child's production of the target behavior as correct or incorrect to determine an accuracy percentage and thus assess improvement over time. It is good practice for the clinician to minimally follow the documentation guidelines dictated by his or her employer.

The clinician can use ***Individual Data Recording Sheet for Multiple Sessions or Multiple Targets*** through ***Therapy Daily Progress Notes/Log*** to record the child's performance in his or her treatment sessions; the forms may be adapted to meet the clinician's and the child's needs.

Probe Recording Sheet may be used during probing procedures to assess for generalized productions of the target sound(s) to other sounds or higher linguistic levels.

Individual Data Recording Sheet for Multiple Sessions or Multiple Targets

Name: _____ Age: _____ Clinician: _____

Date: _____ Target: _____ Accuracy Percentage: ____

Date: _____ Target: _____ Accuracy Percentage: ____

Date: _____ Target: _____ Accuracy Percentage: ____

Date: _____ Target: _____ Accuracy Percentage: ____

Global Data Recording Sheet

Name: _____ **Age:** _____ **Clinician:** _____

Date: _____ **Target:** _____

Accuracy Percentage: _____

Data Recording Sheet for Three Sound Positions

Name: _____ Age: _____ Clinician: _____

Date: _____ Target Sound: _____

Initial Position

Accuracy Percentage: _____

Medial Position

Accuracy Percentage: _____

Final Position

Accuracy Percentage: _____

Group Data Recording Sheet for up to Six Students

Student Name: _____ **Age:** _____ **Clinician:** _____

Target: _____ **Accuracy Percentage:** _____

Student Name: _____ **Age:** _____ **Clinician:** _____

Target: _____ **Accuracy Percentage:** _____

Student Name: _____ **Date:** _____

Target: _____ **Accuracy Percentage:** _____

Student Name: _____ **Date:** _____

Target: _____ **Accuracy Percentage:** _____

Student Name: _____ **Date:** _____

Target: _____ **Accuracy Percentage:** _____

Student Name: _____ **Date:** _____

Target: _____ **Accuracy Percentage:** _____

Data Recording Sheet for 20 Selected Stimulus Items

Name: _____ Age: _____ Clinician: _____

Date: _____ Target Sound: _____ Accuracy Criterion: _____

(+) = correct   (−) = incorrect   (NR) = no response

Target Responses/ Word Exemplars	1	2	3	4	5	1	2	3	4	5	1	2	3	4	5	1	2	3	4	5

Percentage Correct: _____

Progress Summary Graph

Accuracy Percentage ↓ ↓ ↓	Progress Summary Graph CLIENT'S NAME: _____ TARGET: _____																	
100%																		
90%																		
80%																		
70%																		
60%																		
50%																		
40%																		
30%																		
20%																		
10%																		
0%																		
→ Date/ Session # →																		

Sticker Reward Sheet

Name: _____ **For:** _____

Therapy Daily Progress Notes/Log

Student's Name: _____ **Diagnosis:** _____

Clinician: _____ **School:** _____

_____

_____

_____

_____

_____

_____

_____

_____

_____

_____

_____

_____

_____

_____

_____

_____

_____

_____

_____

_____

_____

_____

_____

Probe Recording Sheet

Name: _____ Age: _____ Clinician: _____

Date: _____ Disorder(s): _____

Target Behavior: _____

Target Response	Correct (+)/Incorrect (−)
1.	
2.	
3.	
4.	
5.	
6.	
7.	
8.	
9.	
10.	
11.	
12.	
13.	
14.	
15.	
Percentage Correct	

ESTABLISHING THE PRODUCTION OF SOUNDS

Articulation therapy typically begins by establishing sounds in isolation because children with articulation and phonological disorders often require direct instruction to learn the motor production of sounds. The clinician makes use of special sound-evoking techniques such as phonetic placement, sound approximation, modeling, verbal instructions, and prompts to teach the essential features of the chosen sounds. Some children require modeling to establish appropriate production, while others need more direct manipulation of the articulators. In practice, the clinician generally uses a combination of techniques.

Sound-Evoking Techniques for English Consonants provides sound establishment techniques for all American English consonants. We arranged the sounds according to sound classes and cognate pairs and provided their place, manner, and voicing features along with a review of their articulatory production. The techniques are mere guidelines and should not be considered fail-proof. While one specific technique may work well with a particular child, the same technique may fail with another. Ultimately, it is the clinician's knowledge and experience that help her alter clinical methods to fit the needs of the individual child. See the "Basic Unit" of Chapter 8 in *Assessment and Treatment of Articulation and Phonological Disorders* for more information on the various methods used to establish the motor production of sounds.

SOUND: /p/

Place, Manner, Voicing Features

- Bilabial
- Stop-plosive (aspirate sound)
- Voiceless

Articulatory Production

- Lips are shut lightly.
- Soft palate is raised to assist with velopharyngeal closure.
- Tongue is in a neutral position or in the position required for the next sound.
- Oral (air) pressure builds up behind the shut lips.
- Vocal folds are abducted.
- Lips are separated quickly and breath escapes, creating an explosive sound.

Sound Distribution

- Initial—pig, pot, pin, pen, pass
- Medial—apple, pepper, appointment, apex, appeal
- Final—stop, soup, cape, pop, mop

SOUND: /b/

Place, Manner, Voicing Features

- Bilabial
- Stop-plosive
- Voiced

Articulatory Production

- Lips are shut lightly.
- Soft palate is raised to assist with velopharyngeal closure.
- Tongue is in a neutral position or in the position required for the next sound.
- Oral (air) pressure builds up behind the shut lips.
- Vocal folds are adducted.
- Lips are separated quickly and breath escapes, with less force than for /p/.

Sound Distribution

- Initial—bat, bed, big, be, bay
- Medial—robin, baby, bubble, cabin, pebble
- Final—cab, tub, rib, robe, herb

SOUND-EVOKING TECHNIQUES FOR /p/ AND /b/

Evoking techniques 1–4 facilitate the production of /p/. To establish /b/, follow the same techniques but instruct the child to add voicing or "turn on the voice box." Technique 5 is specific to /b/.

Technique 1

- Hold a piece of tissue paper or other lightweight paper in front of the child's lips.
- Instruct the child, "Close your mouth and fill up your cheeks with air." Provide a model for puffed cheeks.
- Instruct the child to release the air ("blow") and "try to move the piece of paper."
- Draw attention to the force and explosion characteristics of the sound by directing the child's attention to the movement of the paper.
- Gradually shape the amount of air impounded to a more natural level.

Technique 2

- Hold a piece of tissue paper, other lightweight paper, or the back of the child's hand in front of the child's lips.
- Ask the child to repeat "p" in rapid succession.
- Draw attention to the force and explosion characteristics of the sound by directing the child's attention to the movement of the paper or the sensation of air on the back of the child's hand.
- Manually guide the child's lips for adequate seal if necessary.

Technique 3

- Lightly touch the child's upper and lower lips with a tongue depressor or cotton swab stick.
- Ask the child to bring the lips together to touch the spot you touched.
- Place the child's hand in front of the lips.
- Instruct the child to "blow air" through the closed lips.
- Draw attention to the force and explosion characteristics of the sound by directing the child's attention to the "tickling" sensation on the back of the hand.
- Gradually shape the amount of air released by the child.

Technique 4

- Ask the child to kiss the back of his or her hand loudly.
- Draw attention to the lip seal during the kissing motion.
- Ask the child to gradually make the kissing sounds increasingly quieter until they are whispered.
- Instruct the child to remove the back of his or her hand and continue the quiet kisses but to blow air out as the kisses are made instead of drawing air in to "blow the kisses out."

Technique 5

- Ask the child to produce [m] or ask the child, "What sound do we make when something tastes really good? Mmmmm."
- Instruct the child to pinch his or her nose shut while producing [m]; airflow will be forced out through the mouth, resulting in [b]. (Manually pinch the child's nose shut if necessary.)
- Focus the child's attention on the new sound.

SOUND: /t/

Place, Manner, Voicing Features

- Lingua-alveolar
- Stop-plosive (aspirate sound)
- Voiceless

Articulatory Production

- Lips are relaxed and slightly parted.
- Soft palate is raised to assist with velopharyngeal closure.
- Tongue tip and blade are raised to contact the alveolar ridge; the sides of the tongue are raised to contact the upper teeth and gums (forming a seal).
- Oral (air) pressure builds up behind the gum-tongue seal.
- Vocal folds are abducted.
- Gum-tongue seal is suddenly opened and breath escapes, creating an explosive sound.

Sound Distribution

- Initial—tie, top, tub, table, teacher
- Medial—little, after, button, tattoo, city
- Final—cat, act, debt, receipt, quit

SOUND: /d/

Place, Manner, Voicing Features

- Lingua-alveolar
- Stop-plosive
- Voiced

Articulatory Production

- Lips are relaxed and slightly parted.
- Soft palate is raised to assist with velopharyngeal closure.
- Tongue tip and blade are raised to contact the alveolar ridge; the sides of the tongue are raised to contact the upper teeth and gums (forming a seal).
- Oral (air) pressure builds up behind the gum-tongue seal.
- Vocal folds are adducted.
- Gum-tongue seal is suddenly opened, and air escapes with less force than for /t/.

Sound Distribution

- Initial—dog, dad, day, done, double
- Medial—body, fading, daddy, shadow, ladder
- Final—mud, bread, sand, did, could

SOUND-EVOKING TECHNIQUES FOR /t/ AND /d/

These evoking techniques facilitate the production of /t/. To establish /d/, follow the same techniques, but also instruct the child to add voicing or "turn on the voice box."

Technique 1

- Demonstrate for the child the placing of the tongue tip firmly against the alveolar ridge.
- Instruct the child to position his or her tongue tip firmly against the alveolar ridge (a mirror can be used to provide the child with visual feedback).
- Direct the child to hold his or her breath briefly, and then instruct the child to quickly lower the tongue while releasing the breath through the mouth.
- Draw the child's attention to the explosive characteristic of the sound.
- Gradually work to shape the amount of air released in the production of this sound.

Technique 2

- Instruct the child to produce [p].
- Ask the child to position the tongue tip between his or her lips and once again attempt to produce [p]. Now that the child has the sound within the vicinity of [t], he or she will be able to receive both tactile and auditory feedback of a stoplike sound made with the tongue tip.
- Instruct the child to position the tongue tip against the upper lip only and once again attempt to produce a similar sound.
- Instruct the child to make a similar sound with the tongue tip touching the alveolar ridge.
- Note: To evoke [d], develop from [b].

Technique 3

- Place a flavored food upon the child's alveolar ridge by means of a Q-tip.
- Instruct the child to try to remove the food by using the tip of the tongue. Once the child has a "feel" for the position of the tongue tip upon the alveolar ridge, proceed with the following steps.

- Ask the child to position the tongue tip firmly on the alveolar ridge.
- Instruct the child to release the point of contact by lowering the tongue while blowing air out of the mouth.
- Gradually shape the amount of force with which the child expels the air.

Technique 4

- Place a piece of paper or feather in front of the child's mouth just below the upper lip.
- Instruct the child to place his or her tongue tip directly behind the front teeth against the gum ridge.
- Instruct the child to blow air out through his or her mouth while quickly lowering the tongue tip.
- Focus the child's attention on the movement of the paper or feather.
- Gradually, work to shape the amount of force with which the child expels the air.

SOUND: /k/

Place, Manner, Voicing Features

- Lingua-velar
- Stop-plosive (aspirate sound)
- Voiceless

Articulatory Production

- Lips are relaxed and apart.
- Soft palate is raised to assist with velopharyngeal closure.
- Back of the tongue is raised to contact the soft palate, back molars, and posterior gum ridge, forming a seal.
- Oral (air) pressure builds up behind the seal.
- Vocal folds are abducted.
- Tongue–soft palate seal is opened and breath escapes, creating an explosive sound.

Sound Distribution

- Initial—cat, key, kiss, count, quit
- Medial—become, account, cookie, echo, buckle
- Final—back, cake, talk, sick, bank

SOUND: /g/

Place, Manner, Voicing Features

- Lingua-velar
- Stop-plosive
- Voiced

Articulatory Production

- Lips are relaxed and apart.
- Soft palate is raised to assist with velopharyngeal closure.
- Back of the tongue is raised to contact the soft palate, back molars, and posterior gum ridge, forming a seal.
- Oral (air) pressure builds up behind the seal.
- Vocal folds are adducted.
- Tongue–soft palate seal is opened, and air escapes with less force than for /k/.

Sound Distribution

- Initial—go, goat, gate, ghost, girl
- Medial—ego, wagon, burger, magazine, again
- Final—egg, beg, vague, fog, flag

SOUND-EVOKING TECHNIQUES FOR /k/ AND /g/

These evoking techniques facilitate the production of /k/. To establish /g/, follow the same techniques, but also instruct the child to add voicing or "turn on the voice box."

Technique 1

- Instruct the child to position the tongue tip behind the lower front teeth. (If child is unable to hold this position, a tongue depressor may be used to keep the tongue in place.)
- Instruct the child to "raise" or "hump" the back portion of the tongue until it forms a seal with the roof of the mouth (soft palate); oral pressure may be built up behind this seal.
- Instruct the child to quickly break the seal by lowering the back of the tongue and "blowing" air through at the same time, thus expelling the built-up air. Provide a model for visual and auditory feedback.
- Gradually shape the amount of air released by the child.

Technique 2

- Ask the child to produce [t].
- Instruct the child to produce [t] with the tongue tip behind the lower front teeth. With the tongue tip still positioned behind the lower front teeth, proceed with the next step.
- Ask the child to "raise" or "hump" the back of the tongue to the roof of the mouth (the soft palate) and attempt to produce [k]. Provide a model for visual and auditory feedback.
- Note: To evoke [g], develop from [d] instead of [k].

Technique 3

- Instruct the child to produce [i] as in "bee" or "we."
- Instruct the child to produce a prolonged [i] while raising the back of the tongue until it touches the roof of the mouth (soft palate); once a seal is formed, instruct the child

to release the contact. If the resulting sound is more like [g] than [k], instruct the child to turn off his or her voice box or to "whisper" the sound.

Technique 4

- Instruct the child to position the tongue tip behind the lower front teeth. If needed, assist child by means of a tongue depressor.
- Model the production of [k] for the child. If needed, shape your hand like a tongue during the production of [k] in order to give the child some visual feedback for tongue positioning.
- Instruct the child to "raise" or "hump" the back of the tongue to the roof of the mouth (soft palate), forming a seal.
- Instruct the child to allow air to build up behind this seal, and then instruct the child to lower the back of the tongue, thus allowing the built-up air to be released.

SOUND: /f/

Place, Manner, Voicing Features

- Labiodental
- Fricative
- Voiceless

Articulatory Production

- Mandible is retracted slightly as the lower lip is lightly placed against the bottom edges of the upper teeth.
- Soft palate is raised to assist with velopharyngeal closure.
- Tongue is in a neutral position or in the position required for the next sound.
- Vocal folds are abducted.
- Audible friction is produced as air is directed through the upper teeth–lower lip contact.

Sound Distribution

- Initial—feet, fudge, fog, phone, fir
- Medial—elephant, muffin, coffee, aphasia, after
- Final—leaf, laugh, cough, half, roof

SOUND: /v/

Place, Manner, Voicing Features

- Labiodental
- Fricative
- Voiced

Articulatory Production

- Mandible is retracted slightly as the lower lip is lightly placed against the bottom edges of the upper front teeth.
- Soft palate is raised to assist with velopharyngeal closure.
- Tongue is in a neutral position or in the position required for the next sound.
- Vocal folds are adducted.
- Audible friction is produced as air is directed through the upper teeth–lower lip contact.

Sound Distribution

- Initial—vase, verb, vine, vanilla, view
- Medial—television, evil, never, river, seven
- Final—live, love, dove, five, save

SOUND-EVOKING TECHNIQUES FOR [f] AND [v]

These evoking techniques facilitate the production of [f]. To establish [v], follow the same techniques, but also instruct the child to add voicing or "turn on the voice box."

Technique 1

- Instruct the child to bring his or her lower lip in contact with the bottom of the upper front teeth (manual adjustment for adequate contact may be necessary).
- Instruct the child to blow air out of the mouth between the lower lip and the upper teeth. (Make sure there is no voicing added.)
- Have the child repeat this process with a piece of paper or a feather in front of his or her mouth.
- Use the feather or paper to help the child focus on the force of the expelled air.
- Gradually work to shape the force of the expelled air as needed.

Technique 2

- Ask the child to say [ɑ].
- Instruct the child to bring his or her lower lip in contact with the bottom of the upper front teeth while producing a prolonged [ɑ] (if needed, manually guide the child's lower lip up to contact the bottom of the upper front teeth).
- Ask the child to once again attempt to produce [ɑ], this time while blowing air out between the lower lip and upper teeth so that audible friction is produced.
- Instruct the child to repeat the above step with his or her voice box turned off.
- Note: To facilitate [v], ignore the final step of this evoking technique.

Technique 3

- Ask the child to produce [p].
- Instruct the child to produce [p] while moving the lower lip back until it contacts the bottom of the upper front teeth.
- Instruct the child to keep the lower lip in contact with the bottom of the upper front teeth while blowing air out between the lower lip and the upper front teeth so that audible friction is produced.
- Gradually shape the force of the air emitted.

Technique 4

- Instruct the child to "gently bite down" on his or her lower lip.
- Instruct the child to blow air out between the upper teeth and the lower lip. Use a feather or piece of paper positioned in front of the child's mouth to draw the child's attention to the force and direction of the airflow.

SOUND: /θ/

Place, Manner, Voicing Features

- Linguadental
- Fricative
- Voiceless

Articulatory Production

- Lips are relaxed and apart.
- Soft palate is raised to assist with velopharyngeal closure.
- Mandible is lowered slightly.
- Tongue tip is placed lightly behind the upper front teeth, or the blade and tip of the tongue are placed in the space between the upper and lower front teeth.
- Vocal folds are abducted.
- Audible friction is produced as air is directed through the tongue–teeth contact.

Sound Distribution

- Initial—thumb, thigh, thin, thick, theme
- Medial—toothbrush, lethal, nothing, pathetic, healthy
- Final—teeth, truth, both, mouth, beneath

SOUND: /ð/

Place, Manner, Voicing Features

- Linguadental
- Fricative
- Voiced

Articulatory Production

- Lips are relaxed and apart.
- Soft palate is raised to assist with velopharyngeal closure.
- Mandible is lowered slightly.
- Tongue tip is placed lightly behind the upper front teeth, or the blade and tip of the tongue are placed in the space between the upper and lower front teeth.
- Vocal folds are adducted.
- Audible friction is produced as air is directed through the tongue–teeth contact.

Sound Distribution

- Initial—the, this, that, there, then
- Medial—bother, mother, clothing, father, other
- Final—breathe, bathe, smooth, teethe, clothe

SOUND-EVOKING TECHNIQUES FOR /θ/ AND /ð/

These evoking techniques facilitate the production of [θ]. To establish [ð], follow the same steps, but also instruct the child to add voicing or "turn on the voice box."

Technique 1

- Instruct the child to stick his or her tongue "straight out."
- Instruct the child to "gently bite down" on the tongue.
- Instruct the child to slowly retract his or her tongue until only the tongue tip protrudes between the upper and lower front teeth (if needed, assist child by means of a tongue depressor).
- Ask the child to blow air over the tongue and through the constriction formed by the tongue and upper front teeth.

Technique 2

- Ask the child to produce [f].
- Instruct the child to push his or her tongue tip forward between the teeth while producing [f]; this will force the lower lip to release contact with the bottom edge of the upper front teeth, allowing the tongue tip to take its place, thus forming [θ].
- Repeat the previous steps until the tongue protrusion is within normal limits (if needed, manually assist the child with the tongue protrusion).

Technique 3

- Place a tongue depressor or flavored food directly in front of the child's mouth.
- Instruct the child to touch this item with his or her tongue tip; with the child's tongue extended, proceed with the next step.
- Instruct the child to "gently bite down" on the tongue (if needed, manually raise the child's lower jaw so that both the upper and lower front teeth come in contact with the tongue).
- Instruct the child to blow air over the tongue and through the constriction formed by the tongue and the upper front teeth.
- Gradually work with the child to achieve the proper amount of tongue protrusion.

Technique 4

- Ask the child to produce [s]. While the child is producing this sound, proceed with the next step.
- Instruct the child to slide the tongue tip forward until it slightly protrudes between the upper and lower front teeth, thus forming [θ].
- Gradually work to get the tongue protrusion within normal limits.
- Note: For /ð/, shape from /z/

SOUND: /s/

Place, Manner, Voicing Features

- Lingua-alveolar
- Fricative
- Voiceless

Articulatory Production

(Note: This sound may be produced with the tongue in two different positions.)

- Lips are relaxed and apart.
- Soft palate is raised to assist with velopharyngeal closure.
- Sides of the tongue are against the upper molars.
- (a) Tip of the tongue approximates the lower incisors near the gum ridge while the front of the tongue is both raised toward the alveolar ridge and slightly grooved, OR
  (b) Tip of the tongue is narrowly grooved and approximates the upper alveolar ridge.
- Vocal folds are abducted.
- Audible friction is produced as air is directed through the groove in the tongue against the upper alveolar ridge and front teeth.

Sound Distribution

- Initial—city, safe, scent, song, see
- Medial—bracelet, eraser, pencil, proceed, upset
- Final—dance, kiss, jealous, nice, house

SOUND: /z/

Place, Manner, Voicing Features

- Lingua-alveolar
- Fricative
- Voiced

Articulatory Production

(Note: This sound may be produced with the tongue in two different positions.)

- Lips are relaxed and apart.
- Soft palate is raised to assist with velopharyngeal closure.

- Sides of the tongue are against the upper molars.
- (a) Tip of the tongue approximates the lower incisors near the gum ridge while the front of the tongue is both raised toward the alveolar ridge and slightly grooved, OR (b) Tip of the tongue is narrowly grooved and approximates the upper alveolar ridge.
- Vocal folds are adducted.
- Audible friction is produced as air is directed through the groove in the tongue against the upper alveolar ridge and front teeth.

Sound Distribution

- Initial—zoom, zebra, zucchini, zipper, zodiac
- Medial—lazy, dozen, freezer, visit, scissors
- Final—breeze, is, jazz, size, close

SOUND-EVOKING TECHNIQUES FOR /s/ AND /z/

Remember, these sounds can be produced with the tongue tip up or down; therefore, follow the child's lead when deciding which way to teach these sounds.

Technique 1 (Tongue Tip Up)

- Instruct the child to raise his or her tongue so that the sides of the tongue come in contact with the inner surface of the upper back teeth.
- Instruct the child to slightly groove the tongue along the midline. If the child is unable to complete this step, add the following steps: Instruct the child to protrude the tongue and place a drinking straw along the midline; ask the child to slightly raise the sides of the tongue around the straw. Carefully remove the straw from the child's mouth.
- Instruct the child to place the tip of his or her tongue slightly behind the upper front teeth.
- Instruct the child to bring his or her teeth together.
- Instruct the child to blow air out along the groove of the tongue.
- Note: For [z], instruct the child to add voicing or "turn on the voice box."

Technique 2 (Tongue Tip Up)

- Model for the child protruding the tongue slightly between the front teeth as in [θ]; ask the child to position his or her tongue in a similar fashion.
- Instruct the child to blow air over the tongue and through the constriction formed between the upper front teeth and the tongue, thus producing [θ].

- Push the tip of the child's tongue tip inward by using a thin instrument (tongue blade) in order to change [θ] to [s]. Once the child understands the correct positioning of the tongue, proceed with the next step.
- Instruct the child to repeat the steps without your manual assistance.
- Note: To facilitate [z], develop from [ð] or instruct the child to turn on the voice while saying [θ].

Technique 3 (Tongue Tip Up)

- Ask the child to produce [ʃ].
- Instruct the child to retract his or her lips (smile) *and* simultaneously push the tongue slightly forward while producing [ʃ], thus resulting in [s].
- Note: To facilitate [z], shape from [ʒ].

Technique 1 (Tongue Tip Down)

- Instruct the child to raise his or her tongue so that the sides of the tongue come in contact with the inner surface of the upper back teeth.
- Instruct the child to lower the tongue tip so that it is placed behind the lower front teeth near the gum ridge.
- Instruct the child to bring the upper and lower front teeth close together, but not touching.
- Instruct the child to blow air out through the mouth, resulting in [s].
- Note: To facilitate [z], instruct the child to add voicing or "turn on the voice box."

Technique 2 (Tongue Tip Down)

- Ask the child to produce [i].
- Instruct the child to turn off his or her voice box or "whisper" so that [i] is now voiceless. While the child is still producing the voiceless [i], proceed with the next step.
- Instruct the child to gradually close his or her teeth until [s] results.
- Note: To facilitate [z], do not instruct the child to turn off the voice box.

Technique 1 (Tongue Tip Up or Down)

- Instruct the child to place his or her tongue tip behind either the upper or the lower front teeth.
- Instruct the child to draw the tongue tip slightly away from the teeth.
- Instruct the child to close his or her teeth so that they are barely touching (manual guidance may be necessary).

- Place a finger or piece of paper in front of the center of the child's mouth and ask the child to "blow air out over the tongue toward my finger [or the piece of paper]."
- Note: To facilitate [z], instruct the child to add voicing or "turn on the voice box." Shape the level of friction as necessary.

Technique 2 (Tongue Tip Up or Down)

- Place a tongue depressor in the child's mouth against either the upper or the lower front teeth and ask the child to use his or her tongue tip to hold it there.
- Ask the child to keep his or her tongue still while the tongue depressor is carefully removed.
- Instruct the child to close his or her teeth.
- Instruct the child to blow air out, resulting in [s].
- Note: To facilitate [z], instruct the child to add voicing or "turn on the voice box."

SOUND: /ʃ/

Place, Manner, Voicing Features

- Lingua-palatal
- Fricative
- Voiceless

Articulatory Production

- Lips are usually protruded and slightly rounded.
- Soft palate is raised to assist with velopharyngeal closure.
- Sides of the tongue are placed against the upper molars; the tip and blade of the tongue are directed toward the lower front teeth, while the broad front surface of the tongue is both raised toward the hard palate and flattened with a wide groove, thus forming a central opening. This opening is slightly wider and more posterior as compared to /s/.
- Vocal folds are abducted.
- Audible friction is produced as air is directed through the central opening against the palate, alveolar ridge, and front teeth.

Sound Distribution

- Initial—she, shop, sugar, sure, shadow
- Medial—ocean, issue, dishes, fashion, motion
- Final—push, fish, fresh, bush, sash

SOUND: /ʒ/

Place, Manner, Voicing Features

- Lingua-palatal
- Fricative
- Voiced

Articulatory Production

- Lips are protruded and slightly rounded.
- Soft palate is raised to assist with velopharyngeal closure.
- Sides of the tongue are placed against the upper molars; the tip and blade of the tongue are directed toward the lower front teeth, while the broad front surface of the

tongue is both raised toward the hard palate and flattened with a wide groove, thus forming a central opening. This opening is slightly wider and more posterior as compared to /z/.

- Vocal folds are abducted.
- Audible friction is produced as air is directed through the central opening against the palate, alveolar ridge, and front teeth.

Sound Distribution

- Initial—does not occur in English
- Medial—vision, Asia, casual, treasure, decision
- Final—beige, garage, corsage, prestige, camouflage

SOUND-EVOKING TECHNIQUES FOR /ʃ/ AND /ʒ/

Evoking techniques 1–3 facilitate the production of [ʃ]. To establish [ʒ], follow the same techniques, but also instruct the child to add voicing or "turn on the voice box."

Technique 1

- Ask the child to produce [s]. While the child is producing this sound, proceed with the next step.
- Instruct the child to "pucker" the lips while moving the tongue back until [ʃ] results.
- Note: To facilitate [ʒ], develop from [z].

Technique 2

- Ask the child, "What sound do people make when they want to tell someone to be quiet?" The clinician may raise his or her forefinger up to the lips as if making the common symbol for "shhh." This may be enough of a cue to evoke the child's production of [ʃ].
- Shape the sound from this point.

Technique 3

- Instruct the child to raise the sides of his or her tongue so that they come in contact with the inner surface of the upper back teeth.
- Instruct the child to raise the tip and blade of the tongue and place it behind the upper front teeth.

- Instruct the child to slowly slide the tongue along the roof of the mouth to where the bump on the roof of the mouth just begins to go down in the back.
- Once the child's tongue is in position, ask the child to lower the tongue slightly (if needed, direct the tongue down slightly with a tongue depressor).
- Ask the child to keep this position while puckering his or her lips.
- Instruct the child to blow air out through the mouth.

Technique 4

- Ask the child to produce [i]. While the child is producing this sound, proceed with the next step.
- Instruct the child to "tightly pucker" his or her lips.
- Instruct the child to raise his or her lower jaw slightly (manual guidance may be necessary).
- Instruct the child to blow air out while raising the tongue, resulting in [ʒ].
- Note: To facilitate [ʃ], instruct the child to produce [i] with the voice off.

SOUND: /h/

Place, Manner, Voicing Features

- Glottal
- Fricative
- Voiceless

Articulatory Production

(Note: There is no set position for the articulators during the production of this sound.)

- Lips assume the position for the next sound.
- Soft palate is raised to assist with velopharyngeal closure.
- Tongue is in a neutral position or in the position required for the next sound.
- Vocal folds are slightly adducted but not close enough to cause phonation.
- Air is directed through the vocal tract with enough force to produce audible friction.

Sound Distribution

- Initial—who, hat, hurt, heal, honey
- Medial—ahead, rehearse, behavior, lighthouse, behind
- Final—does not occur in English

SOUND-EVOKING TECHNIQUES FOR /h/

Technique 1

- Instruct the child to breathe in through the nose and out through the mouth.
- To direct the child's attention to the emission of the air through the mouth, use a piece of paper placed in front of the child's mouth. Continue to facilitate appropriate loudness and force of the sound by asking the child to "breathe louder."

Technique 2

- Model for the child the taking of a deep breath, holding it, and then releasing this breath through the mouth.
- Focus the child's attention on the sound made as the breath is released.
- Instruct the child to follow the clinician's model.
- Work with the child until the force of air and audible friction are within normal limits.

Technique 3

- Place a feather or paper strip in front of the child's mouth.
- Instruct the child to open his or her mouth slightly and to relax the tongue.
- Instruct the child to attempt to move the paper or feather by blowing air out of the mouth with a bit of force behind it.
- Work with the child to achieve an acceptable degree of force and loudness.

Technique 4

- Instruct the child to part the lips and teeth.
- Ask the child to relax the tongue and lips.
- Instruct the child to cup his or her hand and place it in front of his or her mouth.
- Instruct the child to take a deep breath and then breathe the air out through the mouth into the cupped hand. Focus the child's attention to the feel of the expelled air.

SOUND: /ʧ/

Place, Manner, Voicing Features

- Lingua-palatal
- Affricate
- Voiceless

Articulatory Production

This sound is produced on a single impulse of air

- Lips are apart and either slightly rounded or relaxed.
- Soft palate is raised to assist with velopharyngeal closure.
- Sides of the tongue are against the upper molars, while the blade and tip of the tongue are placed just behind the alveolar ridge, thus blocking the airflow briefly.
- Vocal folds are abducted.
- Airflow is blocked briefly and then audibly released by the lowering of the tongue tip and blade, allowing the air to flow through a broad point of constriction that occurs between the front of the tongue and the alveolar ridge.

Sound Distribution

- Initial—cello, chocolate, cheer, chop, choose
- Medial—nature, ritual, teacher, furniture, virtue
- Final—rich, preach, such, lunch, watch

SOUND: /ʤ/

Place, Manner, Voicing Features

- Lingua-palatal
- Affricate
- Voiced

Articulatory Production

This sound is produced on a single impulse of air.

- Lips are apart and either slightly rounded or relaxed.
- Soft palate is raised to assist with velopharyngeal closure.

- Sides of the tongue are against the upper molars, while the blade and tip of the tongue are placed just behind the alveolar ridge, thus blocking the airflow briefly.
- Vocal folds are adducted.
- Airflow is blocked briefly and then audibly released by the lowering of the tongue tip and blade, allowing the air to flow through a broad point of constriction that occurs between the front of the tongue and the alveolar ridge.

Sound Distribution

- Initial—jam, judge, joke, gentle, gypsy
- Medial—soldier, adjust, magic, religion, tragic
- Final—fudge, edge, image, page, stage

SOUND-EVOKING TECHNIQUES FOR /ʧ/ AND /ʤ/

Evoking techniques 1–4 facilitate the production of [ʧ]. To establish [ʤ], follow the same techniques, but also instruct the child to add voicing or "turn on the voice box."

Technique 1

- Ask the child to produce [ʃ], or to evoke this sound, ask, "What sound do we make to ask someone to be quiet? Shhh!" While the child is producing this sound, proceed with the next step.
- Instruct the child to move the tip of the tongue to the roof of the mouth so that he or she can feel the "bump" behind the upper front teeth.
- Remind the child to "pucker" his or her lips, and then instruct the child to lower the tongue tip while forcing air out of the mouth, resulting in [ʧ].

Technique 2

- Instruct the child to raise his or her tongue tip and blade to the roof of the mouth right behind the upper front teeth.
- Instruct the child to slide the tongue back along the roof of the mouth to the "bumpy" portion of the roof and then the slight decline. Once the child finds the place where the bump begins to decline, instruct the child to keep the tip of the tongue there, and proceed with the next step.
- Instruct the child to "pucker" the lips and to lower the tongue tip while forcing air out of the mouth.

Technique 3

- Instruct the child to place the tip of his or her tongue against the roof of the mouth right behind the two upper front teeth.
- Instruct the child to then slide the tongue tip back slightly to the "bump" on the roof of the mouth. It may be necessary to push the tongue tip back to this position by means of a tongue depressor.
- Instruct the child to "pucker" his or her lips.
- Instruct the child to make the sneezing sound (choo!) by slightly lowering the tongue tip while forcing built-up air pressure out of the mouth.

Technique 4

- Instruct the child to produce the following sentence, in which [t] is followed by [ʃ]: "That ship is at shore?" Other phrases the clinician may use are "what shall," "that shell," "what shape," "that ship." Instruct the child to hold the [t] briefly and then "explode" into the [ʃ], thus forming [tʃ].
- Work with the child to shape the [tʃ] sound from these sentences and phrases.
- Note: To facilitate [dʒ], work from phrases such as "meet you," "had you," "found you," "could you."

SOUND: /m/

Place, Manner, Voicing Features

- Bilabial
- Nasal
- Voiced

Articulatory Production

- Lips are shut lightly.
- Tongue is in a neutral position or in the position required for the next sound.
- Velopharyngeal port is open.
- Vocal folds are adducted.
- Air is directed through the open velopharyngeal port, the nasal cavity, and out the nostrils.

Sound Distribution

- Initial—maybe, mine, me, mud, man
- Medial—lemon, grammar, command, famous, hammer
- Final—calm, home, thumb, jam, dime

SOUND-EVOKING TECHNIQUES FOR /m/

Technique 1

- Instruct the child to bring his or her lips together, breathe in deeply through the nose, and then release the breath out the nose.
- Ask the child to say "Ah."
- Instruct the child to close his or her lips, breathe in deeply through the nose, and then let air out through the nose while saying "Ah."

Technique 2

- Ask the child to take a deep breath through the mouth, close the mouth, and expel the air through the nose. (If working with a very young child, you may take turns doing this with the child so that it becomes more like a game.)
- Instruct the child to repeat the previous step, but also instruct him or her to add voicing or "hum" while expelling the air through the nose.

Technique 3

- Ask the child to produce [bʌ].
- Instruct the child to produce the same sound with his or her mouth closed, letting the air flow through the nose.
- Draw attention to the nasal emission by placing a mirror under the nose.

Technique 4

- Instruct the child to bring his or her lips together and "hum," or ask the child, "What do we say when something tastes really good? Mmmmm!"
- These suggestions may result in the correct production of [m].

SOUND: /n/

Place, Manner, Voicing Features

- Lingua-alveolar
- Nasal
- Voiced

Articulatory Production

- Lips are relaxed and slightly apart.
- Sides of the tongue are against the upper teeth and gums, while the tip and blade of the tongue are raised to contact the alveolar ridge.
- Velopharyngeal port is open.
- Vocal folds are adducted.
- Air is directed through the open velopharyngeal port, the nasal cavity, and out the nostrils.

Sound Distribution

- Initial—name, number, none, knock, knife
- Medial—banana, funny, dinosaur, tunnel, wonder
- Final—sun, can, balloon, skin, listen

SOUND-EVOKING TECHNIQUES FOR /n/

Technique 1

- Ask the child to place his or her tongue in position for [d].
- Instruct the child to close his or her mouth, breathe in deeply through the nose, and hold the breath briefly.
- Instruct the child to let the air out through the nose while attempting to produce [d].

Technique 2

- Instruct the child to produce [ɑ]. While the child is producing this sound, proceed with the next step.
- Instruct the child to raise both sides of the tongue to contact the inner surface of the back teeth and to place the front of the tip of the tongue behind the upper front teeth.

- This should block the airflow through the oral cavity and send it through the nose, resulting in [n].

Technique 3

- Use a visual aid such as a mirror to instruct the child to place his or her tongue tip against the alveolar ridge. With the child's tongue in place, proceed with the next step.
- Instruct the child to breathe in and out through his or her nose.
- Keeping the tongue in position, instruct the child to breathe in through the nose and then breathe out through the nose with the addition of voicing.

Technique 4

- Lightly touch the child's upper gum ridge (alveolar ridge) with a tongue depressor or cotton swab.
- Ask the child to raise the tip of the tongue to contact the spot you touched.
- Instruct the child to breathe in through the nose and breathe out through the nose with the "voice box" turned on.

SOUND: /ŋ/

Place, Manner, Voicing Features

- Lingua-velar
- Nasal
- Voiced

Articulatory Production

- Lips are relaxed and apart.
- Back of the tongue is raised against the lowered soft palate, back molars, and posterior gum ridge.
- Velopharyngeal port is open.
- Vocal folds are adducted.
- Air is directed through the open velopharyngeal port, the nasal cavity, and out the nostrils.

Sound Distribution

- Initial—does not occur in English
- Medial—hunger, stronger, jinx, donkey, singer
- Final—ring, bang, wrong, laughing, evening

SOUND-EVOKING TECHNIQUES FOR /ŋ/

Technique 1

- Ask the child to breathe in and out through his or her nose, and use a mirror to focus the child's attention on the nasal emission.
- Instruct the child to attempt to produce [g] with his or her mouth closed, thus directing the air out of the nostrils and producing an approximation for [ŋ]. Shape as necessary.

Technique 2

- Ask the child to place the tongue tip directly behind the lower front teeth. If necessary, a tongue depressor may be used to keep the tongue in place.
- Instruct the child to "hump" or "raise" the back of the tongue, as in the production of [k] and [g].

- Instruct the child to breathe out of the nose while voicing or with the voice box turned on.

Technique 3

- Instruct the child to produce [i].
- Ask the child now to produce a prolonged [i] while raising the back of the tongue so that it forms a seal with the roof of the mouth, resulting in [ŋ].
- Repeat the above steps while focusing the child's attention on the tongue placement and nasal emission.

Technique 4

- Instruct the child to produce [m], "hum," or attempt to say "ah" with the mouth closed. Choose the method that is easiest for the child—this will allow the child to become familiar with the voicing and nasal emission that accompany this sound.
- Model for the child the tongue position for [ŋ], then instruct the child to "hump" or "raise" the back of his or her tongue while resting the tip of the tongue behind the lower front teeth.
- Instruct the child to once again hum or attempt to say "ah" without moving the tongue from its position, resulting in [ŋ].

SOUND: /j/

Place, Manner, Voicing Features

- Lingua-palatal
- Glide
- Voiced

Articulatory Production

- Lips are relaxed or in the position for the next sound.
- Soft palate is raised to assist with velopharyngeal closure.
- Tongue is shifted forward in the oral cavity and the sides of the tongue are placed against the upper teeth; the tip and blade of the tongue are raised toward the alveolar ridge (approximating the position for /i/).
- The "glide" portion of this sound occurs as the tongue is moved into position for the next sound.
- Vocal folds are adducted.
- Air is directed through the oral cavity.

Sound Distribution

- Initial—yellow, young, year, yogurt, you
- Medial—million, canyon, onion, lawyer, coyote
- Final—does not occur in English

SOUND-EVOKING TECHNIQUES FOR /j/

Technique 1

- Instruct the child to make a quick, tight [ʒ] or to say [ʒ] several times quickly. This will often result in [j]. If not, also instruct the child to slightly lower the tip of the tongue.

Technique 2

- Ask the child to produce [i].
- Instruct the child now to produce a prolonged [i] quickly followed by [u], resulting in [iju]. After the child establishes [iju], proceed with the next step.
- Instruct the child to "make the [i] silent," which will result in [ju].

Technique 3

- Ask the child to produce [ð]. While the child is producing [ð], proceed with the next step.
- Instruct the child to retract the tongue straight back from its starting position until the tip is even with the back portion of the alveolar ridge. Assist the child with retracting the tongue a proper distance.
- Instruct the child to slightly lower the tip of the tongue and continue breathing out with the voice on, thus forming [j].

SOUND: /w/

Place, Manner, Voicing Features

- Bilabial/Velar
- Glide
- Voiced

Articulatory Production

- Lips are rounded and slightly protruded.
- Soft palate is raised to assist with velopharyngeal closure.
- Body of the tongue is moved posteriorly and raised toward the palate while the front of the tongue is placed low in the oral cavity (approximating the position for /u/).
- The "glide" portion of this sound occurs as the tongue is moved into position for the next sound.
- Vocal folds are adducted.
- Air is directed through the oral cavity.

Sound Distribution

- Initial—wood, wire, wake, one, water
- Medial—beware, reward, driveway, power, awhile
- Final—does not occur in English

SOUND-EVOKING TECHNIQUES FOR /w/

Technique 1

- Ask the child to produce [u].
- Instruct the child to produce a prolonged [u] quickly followed by [ə], resulting in [uwɑ]. After the child establishes [uwɑ], proceed with the next step.
- Instruct the child to "make the [u] silent," which will result in [wɑ].

Technique 2

- Instruct the child to raise the back of his or her tongue toward the roof of the mouth, but make sure it does not touch. If needed, assist the child by means of a tongue depressor.
- Instruct the child to round the lips and bring them close together.

- Instruct the child to breathe out while voicing or with the voice box on. Shape as necessary.

Technique 3

- Ask the child to produce [bə] (ask the child to make the sound used to scare someone: "Boo!").
- Instruct the child now to round his or her lips and place them close together.
- Instruct the child to attempt to say [bə] with lips rounded, resulting in an approximation of [bwə]. Shape as necessary.

Technique 4

- Ask the child to produce [u] and [ə].
- Instruct the child to produce a prolonged [u] followed by a quick [ə] while both rounding and placing the lips close together, often resulting in [uwə].
- Instruct the child to "make the [u] silent," which will result in [wə]. Shape as necessary.

SOUND: /r/

Place, Manner, Voicing Features

- Lingua-palatal
- Glide
- Voiced

Articulatory Production

- Lips are usually rounded, or they may take the position required for the next sound.
- Soft palate is raised to assist with velopharyngeal closure.
- Sides of the tongue are against the upper molars, while the front of the tongue is raised toward the palate; tip of the tongue approximates the alveolar ridge (retroflex "r") or points down toward the lower teeth.
- The "glide" portion of this sound occurs as the tongue is moved into position for the next sound.
- Vocal folds are adducted.
- Air is directed through the oral cavity.

Sound Distribution

- Initial—wreath, write, rope, ran, room
- Medial—around, berry, orange, pirate, carrot
- Final—car, appear, chair, core, hair

SOUND-EVOKING TECHNIQUES FOR /r/ AND /ɚ/, AND /ɝ/

Technique 1

- Instruct the child to place his or her tongue tip slightly behind the upper front teeth. Manual guidance may be necessary.
- Instruct the child to "curl the tongue backward" without touching the roof of the mouth with the tongue.
- Instruct the child to round the lips slightly while breathing out with the voice on, resulting in [r] or a close approximation. Shape as necessary.

Technique 2

- Ask the child to produce [ɚ].
- Ask the child to produce [ɚ] quickly followed by a vowel such as [i].

- Instruct the child to produce these vowels together several times, resulting in [ɚri]. After the child establishes [ɚri], proceed with the next step.
- Instruct the child to "make the [ɚ] silent," resulting in [ri].

Technique 3

- Ask the child to place the tongue in position for [d].
- Instruct the child to slightly lower the tip of the tongue.
- Instruct the child to retract the tongue, resulting in the curling of the back of the tongue.
- Instruct the child to slightly round his or her lips while breathing out with the voice box turned on, resulting in [r] or a close approximation. Shape as necessary.

Technique 4

- Ask the child to growl like a tiger ("grrr!"), or ask the child, "What sound does a race car make?" Rrrrr! These cues may result in the correct production of [ɝ].

SOUND: /l/

Place, Manner, Voicing Features

- Lingua-alveolar
- Lateral
- Voiced

Articulatory Production

- Lips are relaxed and apart, or they may take on the position required for the next sound.
- Soft palate is raised to assist with velopharyngeal closure.
- Tip of the tongue is placed in contact with the alveolar ridge, and the sides of the tongue are lowered to create openings on both sides of the tongue.
- Vocal folds are adducted.
- Air is directed around the sides of the tongue as it travels through the oral cavity.

Sound Distribution

- Initial—love, little, leap, lungs, lemon
- Medial—follow, eleven, family, salad, jelly
- Final—ball, fell, shawl, hill, oil

SOUND-EVOKING TECHNIQUES FOR /l/

Technique 1

- Place a tongue depressor under the tip and blade of the child's tongue and lift the tongue tip and blade behind the upper front teeth.
- Instruct the child to breathe out while voicing, resulting in [l] or a close approximation. Shape as necessary.

Technique 2

- Using a tongue depressor, cotton swab, or flavored food, touch the place on the child's alveolar ridge where the tongue tip makes contact for the production of [l].
- Instruct the child to place his or her tongue at the spot you touched. Once there, instruct the child to breathe, allowing the air to flow around the sides of the tongue.
- Instruct the child to turn on the voice box and repeat the previous step.

Technique 3

- Ask the child to produce [ɑ]. While the child is producing this sound, proceed with the next step.
- Instruct the child to slowly lift and place his or her tongue tip behind the upper front teeth, resulting in [l]. If needed, use a tongue depressor to raise the tip of the tongue behind the upper front teeth.

Technique 4

- Ask the child to position the tongue as if producing [ð].
- Instruct the child to lower the jaw slightly.
- Instruct the child to slide the tongue tip up the back side of the front teeth to the alveolar ridge behind the two front teeth.
- Instruct the child to lower the sides of the tongue slightly.
- Instruct the child to breathe out while voicing, resulting in [l].

Source: In addition to the authors' clinical experience, the information for this resource was drawn from various sources, including Bleile (1995), Edwards (2003), Garbutt and Anderson (1980), Medlin (1975), Nemoy and Davis (1980), and Stemple and Holcomb (1988).

USING SPECIFIC TREATMENT ACTIVITIES

Clinicians often use fun and exciting activities to help increase the child's interest and cooperation in therapy. Such activities generally are presented in a game format so the child feels like he is playing rather than working. Though creative and enjoyable activities are essential for all kinds of treatment offered to children, the clinician should carefully structure them so that the child's sound-production training is maximized. The target sounds will not improve if the child spends most of his or her time cutting, pasting, and playing in the absence of production training. Therefore, clinical activities should be planned and organized so that valuable treatment time is not devoted to deciding what to do next; activities should not take more than a few seconds to introduce and initiate.

Sample Treatment Activities includes specific treatment activities that can be used with children of varying ages; the clinician may adapt them as needed.

SAMPLE GAME #1
"LET'S GO FISHING FOR SOUNDS"

1. Cut fish out of poster board or thick paper using a fish pattern. Ten fish may be plenty, but cut out as many as needed.
2. Feed a paper clip through each fish.
3. Write a target sound or word containing the sound on each fish or attach a stimulus picture.
4. Make a fishing pole from a string and magnet (some clinicians purchase a play-size fishing pole that is relatively inexpensive to which they attach a magnet).
5. Place the stimulus items (fish) on the floor and instruct the child to "go fishing" for a word.
6. After the child catches a fish, instruct him or her to say the target sound or word on the fish a predetermined number of times.
7. The child cannot "fish" for another word until he or she successfully produces the sound or target word for the selected number of times.

Suggestions

Avoid giving the child too many choices that could take time from production training. The goal of therapy is to stabilize target sound production, not catching fish. The activity should serve only as a facilitating technique and should not become the target of therapy. One way of preventing this is to lay out one or two fish at a time, rather than all the fish at once. Assist the child in connecting the magnet with the paper clip if necessary.

SAMPLE GAME #2
"LET'S UNCOVER THE PICTURE"

1. Choose a picture of an object such as an animal, superhero character, or cartoon character.
2. Glue the picture onto poster board or thick paper and laminate for multiple uses.
3. "Hide" the picture by taping cut-up pieces of construction paper over the picture.
4. Ask the child to say his target sound, word, phrase, or sentence a predetermined number of times.
5. If the child says the target sound correctly the chosen number of times, he or she is allowed to remove a piece of paper to reveal a part of the picture.
6. The activity continues until the entire picture is revealed.
7. Allow the child to color the revealed picture using dry-erase pens.

Suggestions

The clinician may want to develop a set of laminated pictures that could be reused with multiple children and over various sessions.

SAMPLE GAME #3
"LET'S GIVE IT A SMILE"

1. On a blank sheet of paper, draw 10 faces with eyes, nose, and ears. Omit the mouth.
2. Have the child say the target sound, word, phrase, or sentence a given number of times.
3. After the child produces the target a predetermined number of times, he or she can draw a smile on a face. Continue with the activity until all faces have been given smiles.
4. As an additional reward, allow the child to color the faces and add additional features (hair, neck, cheeks, etc.) when the activity is finished.

Suggestions

The clinician may want to laminate the sheet of faces so that it can be used multiple times and with different children. Different color dry-erase pens can be used to draw smiles and additional features.

SAMPLE GAME #4
"LET'S MAKE A BRACELET"

1. Select medium-sized plastic paper clips of various colors (e.g., blue, yellow, red, white, and so forth).
2. Attach a paper clip to each stimulus card (approximately 10).
3. Instruct the child to select a stimulus card and say the target word a given number of times.
4. When the child produces the target word correctly the determined number of times, he or she can remove and keep the paper clip.
5. As the child "earns" each paper clip, he or she is instructed to connect them, working toward making a bracelet.
6. When the child produces all the stimulus items selected for practice, he or she should have collected 10 paper clips. The clinician can assist the child in connecting the paper clip bracelet around his or her wrist.

Suggestions

If the child is practicing a larger number of stimulus words such as 20, the clinician can help the child make a necklace instead of a bracelet.

SAMPLE GAME #5
"LET'S GO HUNTING FOR EGGS"

1. Photocopy the stimulus pictures selected for training.
2. Fold the photocopied stimulus items and place them inside several (approximately 10) plastic eggs.
3. Hide the eggs around the clinical room area.
4. Make sure to "hide" the eggs in a visible manner so that the child does not have any difficulty finding them. This will ensure that treatment time is not wasted by the activity.
5. After the child finds an egg, instruct him or her to say its target word a selected number of times (e.g., five times).
6. The child must say the target sound correctly the number of times indicated before he or she can find another egg.
7. When the child finds all of the eggs hidden, he or she can be given some playtime or another tangible reinforcer.

Caution

Not all children celebrate Easter; it is important for the clinician to ensure that this activity does not violate the child's cultural or religious beliefs.

SAMPLE GAME #6
"LET'S PLAY BASKETBALL"

1. The clinician can use a clean trashcan or any other container with a large diameter to serve as the basketball "hoop" and several small balls (e.g., 10 balls) to play basketball with the child.
2. Instruct the child to select a stimulus picture card and say the target sound, word, phrase, or sentence a given number of times.
3. After the child correctly produces the target word the predetermined number of times, he or she is allowed to toss the ball into the "basket."
4. When the child tosses every ball into the basket, he or she can be given playtime or another tangible reinforcer.

Suggestions

The clinician should make sure that the ball does not have too much bounce to prevent it from bouncing out of the basket. A foam ball works well. Ensure that the distance between the child and the "hoop" is close enough so that the child experiences success at making baskets.

SAMPLE GAME #7
"LET'S PLAY A MEMORY GAME"

1. Make a photocopied matching set of the selected stimulus pictures containing the target sound (approximately 5 sets for young children and 10 sets for older children).
2. Place the pictures facedown.
3. Instruct the child to pick a card and then to turn over another card in hopes of matching the one picked. The object is to get as many matches as possible. If the second card turned over doesn't match the first card, it is turned back over and left in place. Then the child tries again.
4. Instruct the child to say the target word or the carrier phrase, "I picked the _____" every time a picture is turned over whether there is a match or not.
5. When the child gets all the matches, he or she earns playtime or another tangible reinforcer.

Suggestions

The child and the clinician take turns picking pictures to match. This may make the game more competitive for older children. On the clinician's turn, instruct the child to name the picture or to use the carrier phrase, "You picked the_____."

SAMPLE GAME #8
"LET'S PASTE SPOTS ON THE DALMATIAN"

1. Draw a picture of a Dalmatian dog without any spots. Make several copies of the picture or laminate the picture for multiple uses and with different children.
2. Cut out "spots" that the child can paste onto the Dalmatian or use a dry-erase pen to draw spots on the dog if using laminated picture (cut out at least 20 spots).
3. Have the child say the target sound, word, phrase, or sentence a given number of times.

4. After the child produces the target a predetermined number of times, he or she can paste or draw a spot on the Dalmatian.
5. Allow the child to color the rest of the picture when completed as an additional reinforcer.

Suggestions

The clinician can extend this activity to other common objects such as pasting lightbulbs on a Christmas tree, body parts on a person, spots on a cheetah, spots on a leopard, cherries on a tree, and so on.

SAMPLE GAME #9
"LET'S FEED THE HUNGRY BEAR"

1. Create a bear from a medium-sized brown paper bag.
2. Decorate the bag so that it has eyes, a nose, and a mouth.
3. Create the mouth by making a slit on the paper bag big enough for the stimulus cards to slip through.
4. Ask the child to select a stimulus card and produce its target sound word, phrase, or sentence a given number of times. When the child correctly produces the target the predetermined number of times, he or she can "feed" the bear.
5. The child is then instructed to select another card, and the process is continued until the child has fed all the cards to the bear. When all the stimulus cards are in the paper bag, the child can be given playtime or another tangible reinforcer.

SAMPLE GAME #10
"LET'S HELP THE FROG JUMP AWAY"

1. Make a picture of a frog that can be cut out and laminated for multiple uses.
2. Create a picture of a pond with multiple lily pads forming a path along the pond (draw at least 10 lily pads). Label the first lily pad "Start" and the last one "Finish."
3. Place the picture on poster board or thick paper and laminate for multiple uses.
4. Explain the goal of the game, which is to get the frog to jump his way to the "finish line."
5. Ask the child to select a stimulus card and produce the target sound, word, phrase, or sentence a given number of times. When the child correctly

produces the target the predetermined number of times, he or she can make the frog jump onto the next lily pad.

6. The child is then instructed to select another card, and the process is continued until the child has helped the frog get to the "finish line."

7. When the child has helped the frog reach its goal, give the child playtime or another tangible reinforcer.

USING WORD LIST RESOURCES

When treating articulation or phonological disorders, the clinician often selects words that contain the target sound. With a child who cannot yet read, typical stimulus items are objects or pictures that have the target sound within their names. With a school-age child who has sufficient reading skills, the clinician can use written words as stimuli in addition to pictures or drawings of objects.

Word Exemplar Lists for English Consonants contains a list of words for each English consonant in initial and final position. We separated the words for each sound according to two categories: *simple* and *complex*. The simple word lists consist of CV, VC, CVC, CCVC, and CVCV words. These would be most appropriate for the initial stages of therapy as the child progresses from mastering the sound in isolation and syllables to simple words.

We created the complex words lists to offer a greater challenge for the child who has mastered articulation of a specific sound in words with a simpler structure. At either level, the clinician can also use the word lists to evoke the child's production of the target sound in phrases and sentences by creating a sentence for the child to imitate or by having the child come up with a sentence containing the target word. The clinician may also use the written word lists as a quick resource when simply modeling the word for the child to imitate.

Word Exemplar Lists for English Consonants

Sound	Initial Position	Final Position
/p/		
Simple Words		
	page	ape
	pail	beep
	pass	mop
	pat	cap
	paw	cape
	pay	coop
	pea	chip
	peach	chop
	peck	deep
	peer	gap
	pear	hip
	peek	hop
	peel	hoop
	pick	keep
	pie	lap
	pill	loop
	pole	mope
	pony	lip
	puff	tape
	pull	top
Complex Words		
	pacific	asleep
	pajamas	battleship
	paragraph	buttercup
	peekaboo	cantaloupe
	pelican	championship
	percent	lollipop
	personal	landscape
	pinwheel	hilltop
	pinnacle	flagship
	podium	gumdrop
	pitchfork	ketchup
	politician	round-trip
	peacock	unwrap

Sound	Initial Position	Final Position
	ponytail	teacup
	paintbrush	videotape
/b/		
Simple Words		
	baby	bib
	back	bob
	bad	cob
	bait	crib
	bake	cub
	beach	cube
	bead	dab
	bee	globe
	beep	grab
	beet	job
	bear	knob
	bell	rib
	big	robe
	bill	rub
	bite	sob
	boat	hub
	book	tab
	bug	tub
	bun	tube
	bull	web
Complex Words		
	backache	bathrobe
	backpack	bathtub
	backyard	nightclub
	bandana	sparerib
	banana	ice cube
	bassinet	taxicab
	beetle	wardrobe
	beautiful	cobweb
	beginner	transcribe
	bendable	kabob
	beverage	health club

Sound	Initial Position	Final Position
	bicycle	hot tub
	boardwalk	earlobe
	boom box	lightbulb
	buffalo	doorknob

/t/
Simple Words

Sound	Initial Position	Final Position
	tack	bat
	tag	bite
	tall	boat
	tan	beet
	tell	cat
	tap	coat
	tape	dot
	tear	feet
	ten	gate
	tick	goat
	town	hat
	tip	hot
	toes	hut
	tooth	jet
	top	kite
	tail	eight
	toy	mat
	tub	night
	two	pet
	tea	pot

Complex Words

Sound	Initial Position	Final Position
	tabletop	acrobat
	tapioca	astronaut
	teacher	candlelight
	tangerine	chocolate
	teaspoon	clarinet
	teenager	coconut
	television	doormat
	ticket	grapefruit
	telescope	rowboat
	toddler	nonfat

Sound	Initial Position	Final Position
	toenails	doughnut
	tomato	teammate
	tonsil	sunlight
	toolbox	whole-wheat
	tornado	flashlight

/d/
Simple Words

	Initial Position	Final Position
	dine	bead
	deck	bad
	dome	bed
	day	pod
	deer	cod
	den	food
	desk	feed
	dam	loud
	dice	sand
	dug	hide
	dig	kid
	dip	mad
	dive	made
	dock	mud
	doll	pad
	door	paid
	dot	pod
	dove	red
	duck	read
	dust	ride

Complex Words

	Initial Position	Final Position
	dangerous	arrowhead
	daffodil	gingerbread
	dandelion	battlefield
	daughter	bedspread
	doll house	checkerboard
	dumpling	courtyard
	dandruff	dashboard
	doghouse	hammerhead
	detergent	lemonade

Sound	Initial Position	Final Position
	diamond	masquerade
	designer	mermaid
	dictionary	neighborhood
	doorknob	pyramid
	dinosaur	railroad
	diploma	seafood

/k/
Simple Words

	cab	back
	cage	bike
	cake	beak
	cone	cheek
	camel	chick
	candy	brick
	cuff	cook
	cane	dock
	cap	duck
	cash	flake
	cow	knock
	key	chalk
	kid	lick
	kite	pick
	coat	book
	code	neck
	coil	rake
	coin	rock
	cub	sack
	kiss	tack

Complex Words

	cabinet	backpack
	cafeteria	cupcake
	calendar	artichoke
	caterpillar	broomstick
	cauliflower	camelback
	coconut	diamondback
	coyote	haystack
	cucumber	horseback

Sound	Initial Position	Final Position
	cupboard	snowflake
	kitchen	shamrock
	camouflage	quarterback
	candlelight	racetrack
	cannonball	rattlesnake
	cantaloupe	cookbook
	carnival	turtleneck
/g/		
Simple Words		
	goose	bag
	gate	dog
	gash	fig
	game	flag
	gap	frog
	gas	egg
	gate	hug
	gear	jog
	gecko	jug
	get	leg
	ghost	log
	gift	peg
	gone	pig
	give	rag
	go	rug
	goat	sag
	gold	tag
	golf	twig
	gum	wag
	gown	wig
Complex Words		
	galaxy	bean bag
	galloping	backlog
	garbanzo	bulldog
	gardener	bullfrog
	gumdrop	groundhog
	gasoline	ladybug
	gazebo	litterbug

Sound	Initial Position	Final Position
	gazelle	mailbag
	giggling	pollywog
	goalpost	saddlebag
	goldfish	sparkplug
	golfing	hot dog
	gorilla	chili dog
	gardenia	watchdog
	guitarist	ladybug

/f/
Simple Words

	face	beef
	fig	chef
	fairy	calf
	fall	cough
	fang	deaf
	farm	chief
	feed	half
	feet	hoof
	fence	loaf
	fill	laugh
	film	leaf
	fin	life
	fish	loaf
	fist	cuff
	foam	off
	fog	puff
	foil	thief
	food	roof
	fun	rough
	four	tough

Complex Words

	flamingo	giraffe
	feather	fire chief
	firebrick	dandruff
	football	earmuff
	fourteen	telegraph
	forehead	handkerchief

Sound	Initial Position	Final Position
	footprints	housewife
	firecrackers	sheriff
	fireman	loose-leaf
	fireplace	meatloaf
	fisherman	paragraph
	footstool	handcuff
	flagpole	photograph
	fountain	powder puff
	furniture	stroganoff

/v/
Simple Words

	vast	cave
	vase	cove
	valley	dive
	vein	dove
	veil	drive
	vent	eve
	vest	five
	verb	gave
	venom	give
	veto	grove
	vibe	glove
	video	hive
	village	live
	visa	love
	visit	move
	visor	pave
	voice	save
	volt	shave
	vote	shove
	vowel	wave

Complex Words

	vacancy	adhesive
	vacation	aftershave
	vaccination	beehive
	valedictorian	commemorative
	valentine	decorative

Sound	Initial Position	Final Position
	vandalize	defective
	vaporize	eruptive
	vegetable	evaporative
	ventriloquist	explosive
	veteran	imaginative
	vinegar	locomotive
	violinist	microwave
	vocabulary	negative
	volcano	positive
	volunteer	skydive

/θ/
Simple Words

	Initial Position	Final Position
	thank	bath
	thaw	booth
	theft	broth
	theme	cloth
	thick	earth
	think	faith
	thin	math
	thirty	myth
	thorn	moth
	thud	mouth
	thumb	path
	thump	south
	theory	sheath
	thief	teeth
	thought	tooth
	thatch	both
	thigh	wreath
	thing	Smith
	thong	north
	thimble	breath

Complex Words

	Initial Position	Final Position
	therapy	underneath
	thermometer	bubble bath
	thermos	beneath

Sound	Initial Position	Final Position
	thermostat	birdbath
	thesaurus	blacksmith
	thimble	cheesecloth
	thirteen	fourteenth
	thoroughbred	loudmouth
	thousand	Plymouth
	thunder	tablecloth
	Thursday	thirteenth
	thankful	down-to-earth
	Thanksgiving	washcloth
	theatrical	sixteenth
	therapy	thirtieth

/ð/

Simple Words

	than	bathe
	that	breathe
	the	clothe
	theirs	lathe
	them	loathe
	then	scathe
	there	seethe
	these	smooth
	they	soothe
	this	teethe

Complex Words

	therefore	sunbathe
	themselves	unsheathe
	thereafter	unswathe
	thereabout	unclothe
	thereat	
	thereby	
	therein	
	thereupon	
	thereto	
	therewithal	

Sound	Initial Position	Final Position
/s/		
Simple Words		
	sack	ace
	sad	bass
	sail	blouse
	salt	chess
	same	bus
	sand	case
	sick	dice
	save	face
	sash	house
	seed	gas
	sea	glass
	seal	goose
	soap	dress
	seat	kiss
	suit	lace
	sip	ice
	sob	mess
	sock	mice
	cent	moose
	sun	rice
Complex Words		
	sardine	fireplace
	seashell	birdhouse
	sailboat	wilderness
	sunlight	briefcase
	softball	dangerous
	sausage	colorless
	seasoning	compass
	scissors	toothless
	swordfish	dollhouse
	signature	doghouse
	salami	mattress
	soccer ball	tree house
	sandpaper	necklace

Sound	Initial Position	Final Position
	seventeen	shoelace
	salamander	thermos
/z/		
Simple Words		
	zap	bees
	zinc	boys
	zany	bows
	zebra	eyes
	zero	cheese
	zit	days
	zip	crows
	zone	nose
	zoo	pies
	zoom	hers
	zeal	his
	zippy	hose
	zebu	knees
	zest	fleas
	zombie	shoes
	zinnia	paws
	zing	rose
	zilch	toes
	zeta	toys
	zipped	graze
Complex Words		
	zeppelin	bananas
	zippered	batteries
	zirconium	bumblebees
	zodiac	cranberries
	zoologist	tomatoes
	zoology	dominos
	zucchini	fireflies
	xylophone	sunglasses
	zenith	groceries
	zephyr	potatoes
	zillion	mayonnaise

Sound	Initial Position	Final Position
	zinc oxide	puppies
	zwieback	strawberries

/ʃ/
Simple Words

	Initial Position	Final Position
	shack	ash
	shade	bash
	shaggy	brush
	shape	crash
	chef	crush
	sharp	dash
	shave	dish
	she	fish
	sheep	flash
	sheet	sash
	shell	lash
	shine	leash
	shoe	mesh
	ship	mash
	shop	rash
	shore	push
	short	smash
	shawl	trash
	shape	wash
	shovel	wish

Complex Words

	Initial Position	Final Position
	shattered	airbrush
	shadow	bottlebrush
	shampoo	crayfish
	shamrock	hairbrush
	sharpener	horseradish
	shinbone	mackintosh
	sheepherder	mouthwash
	sheepskin	paintbrush
	shoelace	goldfish
	shopkeeper	rosebush
	shortening	shellfish
	shoemaker	tarnish

Sound	Initial Position	Final Position
	shoulder	toothbrush
	sheepdog	starfish
	shellfish	whiplash
/ʒ/	English words do not begin with /ʒ/ sound	barrage
		beige
		collage
		corsage
		decoupage
		entourage
		garage
		luge
		massage
		mirage
		prestige
		rouge
/h/ *Simple Words*	ham	English words do not end in /h/ sound
	hair	
	hand	
	happy	
	hatch	
	hawk	
	hay	
	harp	
	heart	
	house	
	heel	
	her	
	head	
	him	
	hippo	
	hog	
	hole	
	hose	

Sound	Initial Position	Final Position
	hut	
	hat	
Complex Words		
	helmet	
	hacksaw	
	hammering	
	handbag	
	hammock	
	hallway	
	headboard	
	hamburger	
	hopscotch	
	handkerchief	
	happiest	
	harmonica	
	helicopter	
	headache	
	honeycomb	

/tʃ/

Simple Words

Sound	Initial Position	Final Position
	chain	broach
	chalk	bench
	chap	catch
	chair	couch
	chase	ditch
	child	lunch
	chest	hatch
	charm	hitch
	cheek	hutch
	cheer	latch
	cheese	leech
	cheetah	match
	chess	peach
	chick	notch
	chili	patch
	chin	pooch

Sound	Initial Position	Final Position
	chief	wrench
	chips	sketch
	chew	pouch
	chunk	watch
Complex Words		
	chalkboard	cockroach
	champion	butterscotch
	checkbook	door latch
	ckeckerboard	crosshatch
	chimney	hopscotch
	charcoal	sandwich
	chariot	workbench
	chestnuts	ostrich
	cheekbone	wristwatch
	cheerleader	featherstitch
	cheesecloth	pocket watch
	chimpanzee	approach
	chipmunk	dispatch
	children	top-notch
	chocolate	honeybunch
/dʒ/		
Simple Words		
	jam	pledge
	jacks	badge
	jacket	cage
	jar	bridge
	jelly	edge
	jet	fudge
	jewel	wedge
	gel	hedge
	gym	large
	jade	ledge
	jog	huge
	joke	page
	jaw	judge
	jeep	range
	jeans	ridge

Sound	Initial Position	Final Position
	July	sage
	jug	stage
	jump	wage
Complex Words		
	juggler	cottage
	junkyard	horse carriage
	jaguar	carriage
	jack-o-lantern	backstage
	gentleman	camouflage
	javelin	cartilage
	jackrabbit	village
	gelatin	passage
	journalist	cartridge
	jasmine	luggage
	junkyard	beverage
	gigantic	sausage
	jackpot	plumage
	jellyfish	package
	jawbone	garbage
/w/		
Simple Words		
	one	English words
	wag	do not end in
	watch	/w/ sound
	woods	
	wagon	
	waist	
	worm	
	walk	
	wall	
	wallet	
	wand	
	wart	
	wick	
	web	
	week	

Sound	Initial Position	Final Position
	wing	
	wig	
	wolf	
	wood	
	worm	

Complex Words

	Initial Position	
	waitress	
	walrus	
	warehouse	
	walnuts	
	wildcats	
	waterspout	
	waterfall	
	workbook	
	wilderness	
	workbench	
	windmill	
	wallpaper	
	wardrobe	
	wishbone	
	watermelon	

/j/
Simple Words

	Initial Position	Final Position
	unit	English words
	use	do not end in
	yacht	/j/ sound
	yank	
	yak	
	yam	
	yard	
	yawn	
	year	
	yell	
	yellow	
	yes	
	yet	

Sound	Initial Position	Final Position
	yip	
	yoga	
	yolk	
	you	
	yo-yo	
	yoke	
	unite	
Complex Words		
	yard master	
	unicorn	
	uniform	
	yourself	
	youngling	
	United States	
	universe	
	university	
	utensils	
	yearbook	
	yellowish	
	yesterday	
	youngster	
	yellowbird	
	ukulele	

/l/

Simple Words

	Initial Position	Final Position
	leash	bowl
	lace	ball
	lad	bale
	lady	bill
	lake	smile
	lamb	bull
	lamp	shell
	land	whale
	lane	owl
	loaf	stool
	long	tool

Sound	Initial Position	Final Position
	lime	hill
	lawn	hole
	light	seal
	lid	mail
	lip	pool
	log	mole
	lock	nail
	luck	pail
	limb	school
Complex Words		
	lunchroom	automobile
	lawn mower	basketball
	lagoon	footstool
	landscape	caramel
	ladybug	carousel
	life jacket	eggshell
	locksmith	casserole
	luggage	pinwheel
	lighthouse	ponytail
	lifeguard	nightingale
	living room	racquetball
	leapfrog	buttonhole
	licorice	treadmill
	lumberjack	meatball
	log house	windowsill

/r/
Simple Words

	rat	hare
	rack	bear
	raft	boar
	rag	pair
	ram	stair
	ramp	chair
	rash	wire
	ray	car
	room	door

Sound	Initial Position	Final Position
	ranch	hair
	red	fair
	reef	fire
	reel	star
	ride	oar
	rib	four
	rich	pear
	robe	scar
	rock	mare
	rug	floor
	rose	tire

Complex Words

Sound	Initial Position	Final Position
	raccoon	stoneware
	racehorse	disappear
	rainfall	everywhere
	wrist watch	bookstore
	railroad	handlebar
	rainbow	Labrador
	restaurant	jaguar
	raspberry	candy bar
	rosebushes	drugstore
	recipes	seashore
	rattlesnake	falling star
	referee	dinosaur
	raquetball	nightmare
	rockfish	underwear
	refrigerator	sycamore

/m/

Simple Words

Sound	Initial Position	Final Position
	mouse	beam
	moss	thumb
	mail	comb
	make	chime
	male	dime
	mom	fame
	mole	gum
	March	gym

Sound	Initial Position	Final Position
	mark	drum
	mask	broom
	mat	game
	May	jam
	mop	lamb
	men	lime
	mice	mom
	milk	name
	moose	plum
	moon	ram
	math	limb
	match	swim

Complex Words

	macaroni	ballroom
	magazine	bathroom
	magician	bedroom
	machine	honeycomb
	mustard	classroom
	marshmallow	chrysanthemum
	microphone	coliseum
	microscope	ice cream
	medicine	mushroom
	marbles	dinnertime
	moccasins	bubble gum
	mermaid	monogram
	mosquito	playtime
	motorboat	medium
	mattress	moonbeam

/n/
Simple Words

	knot	bin
	nail	cane
	name	chin
	net	stain
	nap	fan
	neck	fin
	nest	fun

Sound	Initial Position	Final Position
	knob	train
	knee	lawn
	nine	line
	night	spoon
	no	man
	nod	mane
	nose	nine
	nail	pan
	note	phone
	nest	pen
	nun	pin
	nurse	rain
	nut	plane

Complex Words

	Initial Position	Final Position
	kneecap	accordion
	napkins	button
	nightgown	tambourine
	necklace	backgammon
	needlefish	carnation
	nineteen	chameleon
	neighborhood	cobblestone
	newspaper	dandelion
	nightingale	headphone
	noodle	cinnamon
	necktie	submarine
	number	eighteen
	nursery	policeman
	nightmare	telephone
	nostrils	xylophone

/ŋ/
Simple Words

	Initial Position	Final Position
	English words do not begin with /ng/ sound	bang
		tongue
		sling
		ding
		fang

Sound	Initial Position	Final Position
		fling
		going
		hang
		long
		rang
		ring
		sing
		song
		wing
		wrong
		acting
		rung
		gong
		string
		sting

Complex Words

		bowling
		earring
		boomerang
		boiling
		jumping
		camping
		canoeing
		coloring
		car racing
		examining
		exploding
		folding
		gardening
		balancing
		ice skating

USING A MINIMAL CONTRAST THERAPY APPROACH

In the treatment of articulation and phonological disorders, the contrast approaches are most frequently used to increase the effectiveness of a child's communication by establishing the lost phonemic contrasts in his or her speech. These approaches may, however, be integrated into any treatment where phonemic contrasts would improve speech intelligibility.

There are at least three ways in which phoneme contrasts have been used in target behavior selection: *minimal contrast, maximal contrast,* and *multiple contrasts* (see Chapter 7 in *Assessment and Treatment of Articulation and Phonological Disorders* for more information on the similarities and differences between these three methods). In clinical practice, minimal contrasts are commonly called *minimal pairs* because of the stimuli used to facilitate the contrast: written or pictured word pairs depicting the error production and the target production by only one or two contrasts.

Minimal Pairs Word Lists for Common Phonological Processes offers written lists of minimal pair words *(minimal contrast)* for some of the most common phonological processes. The clinician can incorporate these word lists into minimal pair training with children who have appropriate reading proficiency or can use them as a quick resource for the selection of potential minimal word pairs for training. Word pairs are not provided for *maximal contrast* and *multiple contrasts* since the stimulus words or pictures chosen for training always depend on the child's specific sound errors and current skills. Predetermined word lists could not adequately address the child's needs when either the *maximal* or *multiples contrast* approaches are used (see Chapter 7 in *Assessment and Treatment of Articulation and Phonological Disorders* for examples of potential targets).

SYLLABLE DELETION

Definition

Syllable deletion *is the omission of one or more syllables from a polysyllabic word. The syllable with the least stress is the one most often deleted, but deletion of the stressed syllable can also occur.*

Examples

[kep] for **es**cape   [kæn] for can**dy**

[mʌs] for **Christ**mas   [nænə] for **ba**nana

Potential Target Minimal Word Pairs

acorn–corn	address–dress
arrow–air	baby–bee
bacon–bake	barrel–bear
blanket–kit	cranky–key
carpet–car	city–tea
eclipse–clips	elbow–bow
iron–eye	ketchup–catch
helmet–mitt	lion–lie
locket–lock	magnet–net
modem–mode	monkey–key
open–pen	panda–pan
parrot–pair	party–part
peanut–pea	penguin–pen
percent–cent	pillow–pill
pirate–pie	pitcher–pitch
pony–knee	pumpkin–pump
puppet–pet	raccoon–rack
radio–ray	rattle–rat
ribbon–bun	robot–row
rocket–rock	rodeo–road

rooster–stir   saddle–sad
sausage–saw   silo–low
sandwich–sand   spider–spy
spinach–spin   ticket–tick
tiger–tie   zero–row

FINAL CONSONANT DELETION

Definition

Final consonant deletion *is characterized by the omission of the final consonant in a word. This can affect a single consonant or a final consonant cluster, but the entire cluster must be deleted for the error to be classified as a final consonant deletion.*

Examples

[ke] for ca**pe**   [tre] for trai**n**

[mɑ] for mo**m**   [hæ] for ha**nd**

Potential Target Minimal Word Pairs

bake–bay	bead–bee
bite–buy	boat–bow
boot–boo	keep–key
date–day	dime–dye
goat–go	hike–hi
home–hoe	hoop–who
lake–lay	line–lie
load–low	meet–me
move–moo	need–knee
nose–no	news–new
paid–pay	pipe–pie
rail–ray	road–row
sail–say	seat–sea
soap–sew	suit–sue
team–tea	tide–tie
toad–toe	wait–weigh
week–we	zoom–zoo
ghost–go	beast–bee
signed–sigh	count–cow
key–kings	mow–most

CLUSTER REDUCTION

Definition

Cluster reduction *is defined as the deletion of one or more members of a cluster, resulting in a total or partial cluster reduction. In partial cluster reduction, the sounds most often deleted are those that are later developing or those that are more difficult to produce.*

Examples

[pɑk] for park   [tov] for stove

[bu] for **bl**ue   [tæp] for **tr**ap

Potential Target Minimal Word Pairs

S clusters

star–tar	steak–take
spill–pill	spin–pin
spur–purr	spy–pie
scab–cab	scar–car
snail–nail	snap–nap
small–mall	smile–mile
past–pass	scrub–rub
spread–red	spring–ring
cast–cat	feast–feet
ghost–goat	pest–pet

R clusters

brake–bake	bread–bed
breed–bead	brook–book
drill–dill	drip–dip
drive–dive	dry–dye
free–fee	frog–fog
grab–gab	grate–gate
grave–gave	grill–gill

prop–pop	pry–pie
born–bone	heart–hot
carp–cop	part–pot

L clusters

black–back	blow–bow
clap–cap	club–cub
flake–fake	flat–fat
glass–gas	glaze–gaze
plane–pane	plant–pant
play–pay	plot–pot
slip–sip	slow–sew
slash–sash	split–sit
field–feed	cold–code
mold–mode	told–toad

STOPPING

Definition

Stopping *is most frequently defined as the substitution of stops for fricatives and affricates. Although stopping can occur in all positions, it is most commonly observed in the initial position of the word.*

Examples

[pækt] for fact   [bo] for sew

[pe] for say   [pɪn] for fin

Potential Target Minimal Words Pairs for /s/, /ʃ/, /f/

s words

sack–pack	sad–bad
saddle–cattle	sag–bag
sail–pail	sand–band
sandal–candle	sat–cat
saw–paw	sea–tea
seal–deal	seed–bead
send–bend	sew–go
sick–pick	side–tide
sip–dip	sit–pit
bass–bat	chess–check
case–cape	lace–lake

ʃ words

shade–paid	shake–take
shape–tape	share–bear
shave–gave	shed–bed
sheep–beep	sheen–bean
shell–bell	shine–pine
ship–dip	shirt–dirt
shock–dock	shoe–do
shop–pop	shore–tore
shot–pot	show–bow

bush–book	dish–dig
fish–fig	mash–map

f words

face–case	faint–paint
fake–cake	fall–tall
fan–tan	far–car
fast–passed	fat–bat
fell–bell	fig–pig
fin–pin	fine–pine
fish–dish	five–dive
fog–dog	foil–coil
fold–cold	four–pour
beef–beet	deaf–deck
laugh–lap	leaf–leak

Potential Target Minimal Words Pairs for /v/, /ð & θ/, /z/

v words

valet–ballet	van–pan
vandal–candle	vapor–paper
vase–base	veil–tail
vein–cane	vent–dent
venture–denture	verse–purse
very–berry	vest–test
vial–dial	vice–dice
vine–pine	vital–title
volt–bolt	vote–boat
cave–cape	dove–duck
love–luck	shave–shape

ð & θ words

than–pan	thank–bank
that–cat	thaw–paw
theirs–bears	then–pen

there–pear   these–bees
they–day   thick–pick
thin–pin   think–pink
third–bird   thorn–born
those–toes   thought–dot
thread–bread   three–tree
bathe–bake   math–mat
moth–mop   path–pack

z words

zeal–deal   zest–best
zinc–pink   zip–dip
zipper–dipper   zone–bone
zoo–do   zoom–boom
bees–beak   keys–keep
knees–knead   nose–note

DEAFFRICATION

Definition

Deaffrication *refers to the replacement of an affricate with a stop or fricative. Since the affricate class only involves /ʧ/ and /ʤ/, deaffrication can only affect these sounds.*

Examples

[bit] for **ch**eat   [ep] for a**ge**

[dɛk] for **ch**eck   [pæk] for **j**ack

Potential Target Minimal Word Pairs

"ʧ–t" contrast words

chair–tear	chalk–talk
char–tar	chart–tart
chuck—tuck	chatter–tatter
cheek–teak	cheer–tear
cheery–teary	cheese–tease
cherry–terry	chest–test
chew–two	chick–tick
chime–time	chin–tin
chip–tip	chipper–tipper
chop–top	chore–tore
batch–bat	beach–beat
hatch–hat	match–mat
patch–pat	pitch–pit

"ʤ–d" contrast words

gym–dim	jab–dab
jabber–dabber	jam–dam
jangle–dangle	jaunt–daunt
jay–day	jelly–deli
jewel–duel	jig–dig

jingle–dingle

jog–dog

jot–dot

June–dune

badge–bad

hedge–head

page–paid

rage–raid

jock–dock

jolt–dolt

jump–dump

just–dust

budge–bud

ledge–lead

ridge–rid

wage–wade

VELAR FRONTING

Definition

Velar fronting *affects place of articulation through the replacement of the velars /k/, /g/, /ŋ/ with sounds that are made in more anterior positions. The most common substitutions are /t/, /d/, and /n/, although other substitutions can occur.*

Examples

[dɪd] for **k**id	[not] for **g**oat
[ræn] for ra**ng**	[pæt] for pa**ck**

Potential Target Minimal Word Pairs

"k–t" contrast words

cab–tab	cable–table
cake–take	call–tall
came–tame	can–tan
cap–tap	cape–tape
car–tar	coast–toast
cook–took	cool–tool
cop–top	core–tore
corn–torn	cot–tot
back–bat	bake–bait
beak–beat	bike–bite
cheek–cheat	fake–fate
lake–late	like–light
make–mate	rake–rate

"g–d" contrast words

gab–dab	gall–doll
gash–dash	gate–date
gaze–daze	gear–dear
gig–dig	gill–dill
go–doe	got–dot

gown–down

gain–Dane

gust–dust

bag–bad

big–bid

dig–did

mug–mud

sag–sad

game–dame

goat–dote

guy–dye

beg–bed

bug–bud

leg–lead

rig–rid

tag–tad

DEPALATALIZATION

Definition

Depalatalization *is characterized by the substitution of an alveolar fricative for a palatal fricative (e.g., s/ʃ and z/ʒ). Other substitutions within this process include an alveolar affricate for a palatal affricate (e.g., ts/tʃ and dz/dʒ). Others consider any sound change that replaces a palatal sound with a nonpalatal sound as an instance of depalatalization. It is not uncommon for children to replace /ʃ/ with /s/ and /tʃ/ with /t/.*

Examples

[sɑk] for **sh**ock   [tik] for **ch**eek

[fɪs] for fi**sh**   [hæts] for ha**tch**

Target Minimal Word Pairs

"s–sh" contrast words

sack–shack	sag–shag
sake–shake	sale–shale
sallow–shallow	same–shame
sank–shank	save–shave
saving–shaving	sea–she
said–shed	seen–sheen
seep–sheep	seek–sheik
self–shelf	sell–shell
sift–shift	single–shingle
sip–ship	sock–shock
Sue–shoe	suit–shoot
sore–shore	sew–show
sun–shun	Saul—shawl

"t–tʃ" contrast words

tear–chair	talk–chalk
tap–chap	tart–chart
tat–chat	tatter–chatter

teak–cheek	tear–cheer
teary–cheery	tease–cheese
terry–cherry	test–chest
two–chew	tick–chick
time–chime	tin–chin
tip–chip	tipper–chipper
top–chop	tore–chore
bat–batch	beat–beach
hat–hatch	mat–match
pat–patch	pit–pitch

BACKING

Definition

Although not common in normal phonological development, backing may be observed in children with severe phonological disorders. This process is the opposite of velar fronting and occurs when sounds with an anterior point of constriction are replaced by posterior sounds.

Examples

[ku] for **t**o   [gor] for **d**oor

[pʊk] for pu**t**   [bæg] for ba**d**

Potential Target Minimal Word Pairs

"t–k" contrast words

tab–cab	table–cable
take–cake	tall–call
tame–came	tan–can
tap–cap	tape–cape
tar–car	toast–coast
took–cook	tool–cool
top–cop	tore–core
torn–corn	tot–cot
bat–back	bait–bake
beat–beak	bite–bike
cheat–cheek	fate–fake
late–lake	light–like
mate–make	rate–rake

"d–g" contrast words

dab–gab	doll–gall
dash–gash	date–gate
daze–gaze	dear–gear
dig–gig	dill–gill

doe–go	dot–got
down–gown	Dane–gain
dame–game	dote–goat
dust–gust	dye–guy
bad–bag	bed–beg
bid–big	bud–bug
did–dig	lead–leg
mud–mug	rid–rig
sad–sag	tad–tag

LIQUID GLIDING (w–r, w–l)

Definition

Liquid gliding *is defined as the substitution of a glide for a prevocalic liquid. This process affects manner of articulation.*

Examples

[wɑk] for **r**ock	[wæp] for **l**ap
[wɪp] for **r**ip	[wæf] for **l**augh

Potential Target Minimal Word Pairs

"w–r" contrast words

wad–rod	waste–raced
wag–rag	wage–rage
wail–rail	whale–rail
wake–rake	wear–rare
way–ray	wed–red
week–reek	went–rent
wide–ride	wig–rig
wing–ring	wink–rink
whip–rip	wise–rise
walk–rock	won–run
want–runt	what–rut

"w–l" contrast words

waste–laced	wag–lag
where–lair	wake–lake
wait–late	waiter–later
wax–lax	way–lay
wean–lean	weave–leave
wed–led	wedge–ledge
week–leek	wept–leapt
wide–lied	why–lie
whip–lick	wick–lick
wilt–lilt	wine–line
wink–link	whip–lip
wizard–lizard	walk–lock
watt–lot	went–lent

TRAINING "R" AND ITS MANY ALLOPHONES

Training "r" with some children can be extremely challenging. Many clinicians can attest to the tremendous amount of work and patience it can take to establish and maintain correct "r." It is not uncommon for some children to receive speech and language services for "r" production for many years from initial diagnosis at 7 or 8 years well into the middle-school years and beyond. This situation can be frustrating for the child, his or her parents, and the clinician.

One of the difficulties with training "r" is that unlike other consonants, this sound has a great number of allophonic variations that may fall under different response classes. These variations result from the surrounding phonetic context such as the preceding or following vowel. It is not uncommon for the clinician to establish production of "r" in one phonetic context only to have the child's production fall apart in another context. For example, the child may produce "r" in initial position preceding /i/ and /ɪ/ yet have continued difficulties with its production in all other contexts. The same may hold true for stressed and unstressed "er."

Because of the complexity of this sound, the clinician should never assume that teaching "r" and "er" in one context will lead to generalized productions to other contexts, which can only be ascertained by continual *probing* procedures. Rather than developing a broad goal of "r" and "er" at specific levels of training, the clinician should narrow the target objective to the specific phonetic context(s) in which the child is expected to acquire production. A typical treatment goal statement such as "the production of 'r' in initial, medial, and final position at the sentence level with 90% accuracy across three clinical sessions" may be too general. Rather, the clinician may need to write objectives that outline the specific phonetic context(s) chosen for training such as, "the production of prevocalic 'r' with 90% accuracy in words followed by the vowels /æ/, /ɑ/, and /e/." The clinician could then assess for generalized productions to other contexts such as /i/, /ɪ/, /ɛ/ and train if necessary.

Prevocalic, Postvocalic, and Syllabic "R" Word Lists contains possible target words, selected and organized for consonantal and syllabic "r" in three major groups: *prevocalic, postvocalic,* and *stressed and unstressed syllabic "r."* This resource can help the clinician identify potential target words for training "r" in specific phonetic contexts.

"R" Production Word Cue Cards provides cue cards that correspond to "r" in the postvocalic and syllabic phonetic contexts outlined in the "R" Word Lists resource.

PREVOCALIC "R" GROUP

"A" Subgroup

/r/ precedes vowel: /e/

rabies	race	racecourse
racehorse	rate	racetrack
racial	racism	radar
radial	radiant	radiate
radiation	radiator	radio
radius	rage	raid
rail	railing	railroad
rain	rainbow	raincoat
raindrop	rainstorm	raise
raisin	rake	ramie

/r/ precedes vowel: /æ/

rabbet	rabbit	rabble
rabid	raccoon	rack
racket	racketeer	racquetball
radical	radish	raffia
raffle	raft	rag
ragamuffin	ragged	ragweed
rally	ram	ramble
rambler	rambunctious	ramp
rampage	ran	ranch
rancid	random	rang
rhapsody	wrack	wrangle
wrap	wrapper	wrath

"E" Subgroup

/r/ precedes vowel: /ɛ/

readily	ready	realm
rebel (noun)	recipe	reckless
reckon	reckoning	recluse
recognition	recognize	recollect
recommend	recompense	reconcile
record (noun)	recognize	rent
recreate (verb)	rectangle	rectify
rectitude	recto	rector
red	redden	reddish
red-handed	redhead	red-hot
redwood	referee	refuge
wreck	wreckage	wren
wrench	wrestle	wretch

/r/ precedes vowel: /i/

reach	react	read
reading	reagent	real
reality	ream	reap
reason	reassure	rebate
rebound	rebus	recap
recent	recess	reconsider
reconstruct	reed	reef
reek	reel	reentry
refill	reflex	reflexive
regency	regent	region
wreak	wreath	wreathe

/r/ precedes vowel: /ɪ/

rebel (verb)	rebellion	rebellious
rebuff	rebuke	rebuttal
recall	recant	recede
receipt	receive	receiver

receptacle	reception	receptionist
receptive	receptor	recession
recessive	recipient	reciprocal
reciprocate	recital	recite
reclaim	recline	recoil
record (verb)	recorder	recording
recount (verb)	recoup	recover

"ɪ" Subgroup

/r/ precedes vowel : /ɪ/

rhythm	rib	ribbon
rich	Rick	riches
rickets	ricochet	ricotta
rickety	Richter scale	riches
rid	riddle	ridge
rift	rig	rigid
rigor	ring	rink
rinse	rip	ripple
wriggle	wring	wrinkle

/r/ precedes diphthong: /ai/

rhinestone	rhino	rice
ride	rider	rife
right	right-hand	rhyme
riot	ripe	rise
rite	rival	rive
write	writer	write-up
write-in	writhe	writing

"O" Subgroup

/r/ precedes vowel: /a/

rhombus	rob	robin
rock	rocker	rocket

rocky	rod	roger
rollick	romp	romper
roster	rot	rotten
wrong	wrongdoer	wrongful
wrought	wrought iron	wroth

/r/ precedes vowel: /o/

roach	road	roadblock
roam	roast	robe
robot	robust	rode
rodent	rodeo	rogue
role	Roman	Rome
romance	romantic	rope
rose	rosebud	rosebush
rosewood	rosy	rote
wrote	rotate	rotund
rotunda	rotation	rotisserie
rove	row	wrote

/r/ precedes vowel: /u/

rheumatic	rood	roof
roofing	room	roommate
roost	rooster	root
rouge	roulade	roulette
route	routine	rube
rubella	rubric	ruby
rude	rudiment	rue
ruin	rule	ruler

/r/ precedes vowel: /oi/

| roil | royal | royal blue |
| royalist | | |

/r/precedes vowel: /au/

round	roundabout	roundhouse
roundly	rouse	rout
roundup	round-the-clock	rowdy

"U" Subgroup

/r/ precedes vowel: /ʌ/

rough	roughage	roughhouse
roughneck	rub	rubber
rubberneck	rubber-stamp	rubbing
rubbish	rubble	rubdown
ruckus	ruddy	ruffle
rug	rugby	rugged
rumba	rumble	rummage
rummy	rump	run
runaway	run-down	rung
runner	runny	runt
runway	rupture	rush
rust	rut	wrung

POSTVOCALIC "R" GROUP

"ar"—/r/ follows vowel: /ɑ/

Initial Position

arbor	arc	arcade
arch	archery	arches
arcs	arctic	are
ardent	armful	argue
ark	arm	armpit
armor	army	Arnold
art	Arthur	artist

Medial Position

alarm	barbell	barber
sharpen	bark	barn
park	barnyard	bars
card	cardboard	carpet
cars	chart	dark
darts	farm	hard
mark	part	shark

Final Position

ajar	are	bar
bizarre	car	crowbar
far	guitar	jar
mar	par	our
racecar	radar	sandbar
scar	sonar	spar
star	toolbar	tar

"or"–/r/ follows vowel: /o/

Initial Position

oral	orange	orb
orbit	orchard	orchestra
orchid	ordeal	order
ordinary	ornament	Oregon
orator	organ	organize
orient	origin	ordain
oracle	orphan	organic

Medial Position

accordion	coral	cord
cork	corn	corner
doorbell	florist	foreign
forest	fork	fort
gorge	horn	horse
north	popcorn	score
short	snore	torch

Final Position

adore	ashore	before
boar	chore	core
door	floor	your
four	more	oar
pour	roar	score
shore	snore	sore
store	tore	wore

"air"–/r/ follows vowel: /ɛ/

Initial Position

aerate	aerial	aerosol
air	airbrush	aircraft
airline	airmail	airplane
airport	airtight	area
aerobics	airsick	airline
airbag	airway	aerospace

Medial Position

barefoot	bareback	barely
bare	careless	caretaker
carefree	chairman	chairs
dairy	fairground	fairy
fairytale	hairball	hairdryer
haircut	hare	stairs
staircase	naris	harelip

Final Position

bear	camel hair	care
chair	dare	fair
flare	hair	lair
millionaire	pear	despair
rare	repair	scare
share	square	stare
wear	tear	unfair

"ear" "eer"–/r/ follows vowel: /i/

Initial Position

ear	earache	eardrum
earlobe	earmark	earmuffs
earplugs	earring	earwax
earphone	earshot	earwig
earsplitting	eerie	earflap

Medial Position

beard	bleary	cheerful
cheerleader	cheers	clearance
dearest	gears	dreary
hearing	hero	nearby
hearsay	spearfish	spears
steered	tears	weary
yearbook	yearly	fearless

Final Position

appear	clear	deer
disappear	fear	spear
gear	peer	headgear
hear	midyear	near
overhear	reappear	rear
sear	shear	smear
tear	unclear	year

"irr"–/r/ follows vowel: /ɪ/

Initial Position

Iroquois	irrecoverable	irremediable
irremissible	irremovable	irreplaceable
irrepressible	irreproachable	irresistible
irrespective	irresponsible	irretrievable

irreverence	irreversible	irrigable
irrigate	irritable	irritant
irritate	Iroquoian	irreligious

"ire"–/r/ follows the diphthong: /ai/

Initial Position

ire	Ireland	iron

Medial Position

attired	admired	expired
fireball	firebug	firecracker
fired	firefighter	firefly
firehouse	fireman	fires
fireworks	hired	perspired
required	tired	tires
umpiring	wired	wireless

Final Position

acquire	admire	afire
attire	backfire	bonfire
campfire	empire	entire
expire	fire	mire
haywire	hire	liar
require	retire	tire
umpire	vampire	wire

"ure –/r/ follows diphthong: /ju/

Medial Position

cure all	curettage	curia
curie	curio	curious
bureau	bureaucracy	burette

furious	furor	Huron
mural	purebred	puree
purify	purism	Puritan
security		

Final Position

cure	demure	secure
pure	procure	

STRESSED AND UNSTRESSED SYLLABIC "R" GROUP

"ir"

Initial Position /ɝ/

irk   irksome

Medial Position /ɝ/

birth	birch	bird
birthday	circle	circus
circuit	chirp	confirm
dirt	firm	first
gird	shirt	skirt
skirmish	smirk	squirm
squirt	stirring	stirrup

Final Position /ɝ/

fir	sir	stir
whir		

"ur"

Initial Position /ɝ/

Ur	urban	urbanize
urchin	urd	urge
urged	urgent	urn

Medial Position /ɝ/

adjourn	auburn	blurred
blurry	blurb	blurt
burden	burger	burglar
burn	burp	burro
curb	curd	curry
cursive	cursor	curt
curtain	curve	unhurt

Final Position /ɚ/ and /ɝ/

Arthur	assure	blur
brochure	burr	capture
creature	flour	fur
furniture	hour	measure
nature	pasture	our
picture	purr	scour
sour	spur	sure

"er" "ear"

Initial Position /ɝ/

ergo	ergot	ermine
earl	early	earn
earth	earthquake	earthworm
earnest	earning	earthly
earthen	earthenware	earthling
earthshaking	earthward	earthy

Medial Position /ɚ/ and /ɝ/

advertise	afternoon	battery
bakery	fern	delivery
desert	elderly	emergency
energy	bitterness	fingernail
groceries	germs	herd
hibernate	jerky	lantern
liberty	mermaid	pattern

Final Position /ɚ/

blender	brother	dancer
farmer	father	hammer
hanger	hiker	jogger
juggler	mother	November
number	over	pepper
rooster	smaller	softer
taller	tiger	toaster

"rl"

Initial Position /ɝl/

earl

Medial Position /ɝl/

curled	curls	furled
girlfriend	gnarled	girlish
girlhood	girlishness	girlishly
hurled	pearls	swirled
twirled	whirlpool	world
worldly	whirled	snarled

Final Position /ɝl/

burl	curl	furl
girl	hurl	pearl
gnarl	snarl	swirl
twirl	whirl	squirrel

"ar"

Key Words:

Initial
art

Medial
cart

Final
far

"or"

Key Words:

Initial
orchid

Medial
boring

Final
shore

"air"

Key Words:

<u>Initial</u>　　　**<u>Medial</u>**　　　**<u>Final</u>**
airline　　　fair　　　chair

"ear"

Key Words:

<u>Initial</u>　　　**<u>Medial</u>**　　　**<u>Final</u>**
earplug　　　yearly　　　fear

"irr"

Key Words:

Initial
irritate

"ire"

Key Words:

Initial   **Medial**   **Final**
Ireland   fired   tire

"ure"

Key Words:

Initial

- - - - - - - - -

Medial
curio

Final
secure

"er"

Key Words:

Initial
ermine

Medial
fern

Final
her

"ir"

Key Words:

Initial
irk

Medial
bird

Final
fir

"ur"

Key Words:

Initial
urban

Medial
hurt

Final
fur

"rl"

Key Words:

Initial	**Medial**	**Final**
earl	curled	girl

INVOLVING THE CHILD'S PARENTS AND FAMILY IN THERAPY

With close guidance by the clinician, parents and significant others can become an integral part of a child's articulation and phonological training. After the sound or target skill has been well established, the clinician can train parents to identify the desirable and undesirable productions, evoke target skills by modeling and giving verbal and visual instructions, provide subtle prompts such as hand signals to facilitate correct productions, reinforce correct productions, provide corrective feedback for incorrect productions of the target sounds through subtle signals, stop reinforcing incorrect productions, and conduct home treatment programs after adequate training by the speech–language pathologist.

The extent to which parents participate in therapy varies widely. Some parents take a keen interest in their children's treatment and are willing and ready to do anything possible to help. Other parents may not seem quite as interested. However, parents who appear disinterested often do not realize that they have a role in therapy until the clinician makes them aware of such. The clinician should not assume that parents are disinterested until all attempts have been made to involve them in therapy. If a parent continues to refuse to extend therapy into the home environment, the clinician should, in a candid yet supportive way, make it clear that it could limit the child's overall progress in therapy.

At all stages of treatment, the clinician should be careful not to give assignments that may prove detrimental to the child-parent relationship by placing unnecessary tension during home practice. For example, the clinician should not expect parents to facilitate correct production of a sound at home if the sound has not been well established in the therapy setting. It would be counterproductive to expect a child and parent to practice "r" at home if the child's production accuracy level is very low in the clinical setting. Home practice should serve as a reinforcing activity that helps strengthen and maintain a skill that is already produced with high accuracy in the speech therapy room.

The clinician may use ***Letter to Parents for Suggested Speech Therapy Activities at Home*** and ***Tally Form for Home Practice*** as a handout for parents at the appropriate stages of treatment. We recommend that the clinician edit the letter to make it personal; the child's name should be preferred to the pronouns used in the sample.

Letter to Parents for Suggested Speech Therapy Activities at Home

Dear Parents,

    As you know, _____ has been practicing the following sounds / skills in speech therapy:

_____

_____

To improve _____'s chances of using the sound in environments other than the speech room, it is very important that you devote at least a few minutes out of each day to practice with [*him or her*]. I know that your day is very busy, but ongoing practice at home may help your child make faster and more stable progress in his articulation and phonological skills. The following is a list of ideas on how to practice at home. This list is not exhaustive and you can alter it to accommodate your family's routine.

Activities for sound at word, phrase, and sentence levels (have your child practice his or her sound at the current level of practice): _____

1. Read with [*name*] at least once a day for approximately 15–20 minutes. After your child is done practicing [*his or her*] oral reading for the day, go back to the beginning of the story and play a "word search" game. Help your child find at least 15 words that begin or end with [*his or her*] sound and then instruct [*him or her*] to make the sounds using her "best speech." As described later in this letter, give your child specific feedback as needed.

2. Take the Sunday newspaper ads or a magazine and play a treasure hunt game. Help [*name*] find 10–20 advertised objects that have [*his or her*] sound in the word and make a written list of the words, circle the objects, or cut them out and place them on 3 × 5 index cards. Instruct your child to produce the sounds using [*his or her*] "best speech." Give [*name*] specific feedback as needed.

3. During a ride in the car, play a "sound hunting" game. As you drive, have [*name*] find objects that have [*his or her*] sound in them. Offer your child specific feedback as needed. Take turns finding objects. When you find an object that has your child's sound, encourage [*him or her*] to say the word along with you.

4. Go for a "treasure sound hunt" around the house or a particular room and look for things that start or end with the sound that [*name*] is working on. Instruct your child to produce the sounds using his "best speech." Offer your child specific feedback as needed.

5. Create a family fun night or day by playing a board game or a card game. Follow the rules of the game with one slight alteration. As [*name*] is up for a turn, ask [*him or her*] to say a word that contains [*his or her*] sound. If your child does not think of a word in a timely

manner, help [*him or her*] as needed. Offer your child specific
feedback as needed.

6. Play a guessing game in which you think of a word containing your child's
target sound and you provide clues to help [*him or her*] guess the word.
Keep the words and clues simple so that most of the time is devoted to
practicing the sound rather than coming up with the word. Take turns
guessing and giving clues. Offer [*name*] specific feedback as needed.

Activities to promote use of target sound in connected speech activities such as reading and oral conversation.

1. At least 2–3 times per week, have [*name*] give you a synopsis of [*his or her*] school day activities while paying close attention to the production of [*his or her*] target sound(s).
2. During daily reading homework, have [*name*] read aloud for at least 3–5 minutes while paying close attention to the productions of [*his or her*] target sound(s).
3. Read a story to [*name*] and have [*him or her*] summarize it, paying close to the production of [*his or her*] target sound(s).

During home speech practice, please give [*name*] very specific feedback about [*his or her*] productions. Please keep your comments extremely positive. If you notice that [*name*] is producing the target sounds correctly, offer such feedback as, "Sammy, you are doing such a nice job making your 'r' sound. I am noticing a lot of improvement with your practice." If you notice incorrect productions, offer such comments as, "Boy, Tina, I really like how hard you are working on your sound. As you've been reading, though, I've noticed that your tongue is sticking out a bit as you make your 's'. Try putting your tongue back so that your 's' sounds crisper." You can use the attached tally forms to record your child's performance. Please make sure that you give more positive feedback (verbal praise) than corrective feedback to your child. This means that you should more often catch [*name*] producing the target sounds correctly than incorrectly.

Never embarrass [*name*] in front of [*his or her*] friends, relatives, or other important people in [*his or her*] life by correcting productions during social activities. It is better if you and your child develop a nonverbal signal that can be used inconspicuously while out in public. For example, a light squeeze of the shoulder may signal your child that [*he or she*] needs to watch [*his or her*] sound productions as [*he or she*] is talking. Try to signal during a natural break rather than when [*name*] is in the middle of communicating an important thought. Practice these types of signals at home to ensure better success in outside situations.

Thank you so much for your help,

_____
Speech–Language Pathologist

Tally Form for Home Practice

Dear Parents,

Please use the attached *tally form*(s) to record your child's productions during speech practice at home. Send the form(s) back to the speech room with your child every _____. I will review these forms with your child during therapy time and send some new forms home. Thank you so much for helping your child practice the target speech sounds. Your effort will be rewarded by improved speech in important settings like home. Don't worry if you do not record all productions. Do the best that you can. The most important part of this exercise is that your child knows that you are also listening for improvement in his or her target sounds.

TALLY FORM

Target sound: _____ **Level of practice:** _____

Return date: _____ (+) = correct (−) = incorrect

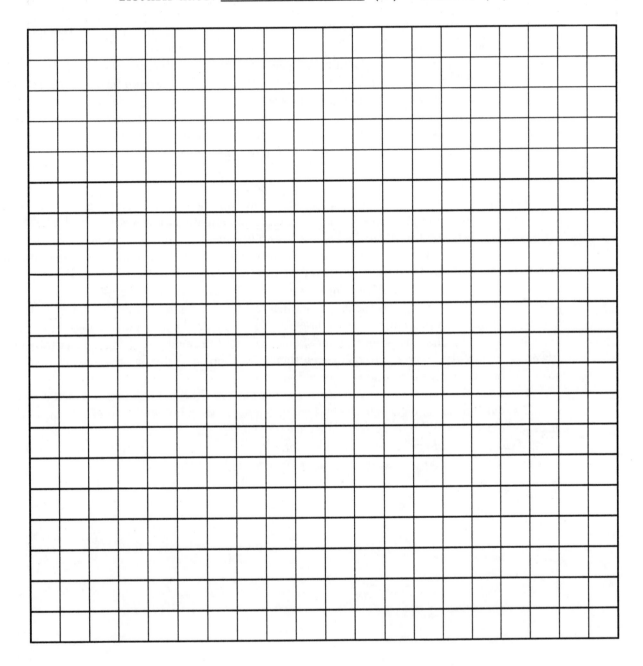

WORKING WITH CLASSROOM TEACHERS

Classroom teachers play a significant role in children's lives. Children are in school an average of 7 hours a day, and the majority of that time is spent interacting with the classroom teacher. The child with an articulation disorder is no exception. Therefore, if the articulation and/or phonological skills trained by a speech–language pathologist are to be maintained in the child's natural environments, it is important that the classroom teacher become an integral part of therapy. We have found that most classroom teachers are willing to help "in some way."

In our delivery of articulation and phonological treatment, we have found that the teacher's role is most significant in the maintenance phase of therapy. After a sound has been well established and the child can produce it consistently at least at the sentence level, it is wise to train the classroom teacher to provide corrective feedback and reinforcement for the child's productions. Teachers can also be asked to give the child specific cues to help improve the production of the target sound in the classroom. For example, the teacher may be trained to instruct the child, "Emily, remember to put your tongue behind your teeth when you make your 's' sound." Nonverbal cues such as hand signals may also be used in the classroom.

The clinician can suggest to the classroom teacher that he or she discuss the importance of speech therapy with the child to encourage the child to regularly attend sessions and take them seriously. Teachers can be encouraged to ask the child what types of activities he or she does in speech therapy. The clinician can also coordinate services with the classroom teacher so that classroom materials are used in the speech therapy room. This will aid in the generalization and maintenance of learned skills. For example, the clinician may have the child practice an assigned oral presentation in the speech therapy room before he or she is scheduled to deliver it in the classroom. Classroom vocabulary and spelling word lists may also be incorporated into the therapy session. Minimally, the classroom teacher should be kept informed of the reason that the child leaves his or her classroom to attend speech therapy sessions and should be made aware of the goals and objectives that the child is expected to achieve.

Confidential Information Handout for Classroom Teachers can be completed by the school-based clinician and given to the classroom teacher to keep him or her abreast of the child's goals and objectives in the speech and language program.

"Tips for Teachers" Letter includes some general suggestions as to how the classroom teacher can help a child with a speech and or language delay in the classroom setting.

Confidential Information Handout for Classroom Teachers

Dear _____,

      The following child in your class has an established Individualized Education Program (IEP) under the speech and language program: _____. It is important that you are aware of this information so that necessary accommodations are made to the student's regular education curriculum. Please note that this information is extremely confidential and should not be shared with uninterested parties.

      The current IEP was established on: _____

      The expected date for review is: _____

The following speech and language goals were agreed upon at the IEP meeting:

1. _____

   _____

   _____

2. _____

   _____

   _____

3. _____

   _____

   _____

4. _____

   _____

   _____

5. _____

   _____

   _____

Please note the following regular education accommodations needed to promote your student's success in the classroom:

1. _____

   _____

   _____

2. _____

_____

_____

3. _____

_____

_____

Other ways that you could help your student achieve his speech–language therapy goals include:

1. _____

_____

_____

2. _____

_____

_____

3. _____

_____

_____

Thank you for your support in this matter. I look forward to collaborating with you, as I believe that you are an integral part in the student's progress. Please feel free to call or e-mail me if you have any questions. You can locate me in Rm. _____. My phone extension is _____. My e-mail address is _____.

_____

Speech–Language Pathologist

"Tips for Teachers" Letter

Dear Classroom Teacher,

As you know, _____ has an active Individualized Education Program due to speech and language difficulties. I would like you to know that I value the positive influence that you have on all of your students, including _____. You are an integral part of the team in helping _____ achieve his/her speech and language goals and to become a better communicator. Unfortunately, for some children, attending speech and language sessions can be a source of distress or embarrassment. Many children with speech and language difficulties are teased, and this can create an emotional sensitivity to anything related to speech and language. I believe that as _____'s classroom teacher, you can help him/her develop a very positive outlook toward the speech and language program and his/her role in the program. Below are some general tips that you may use to help _____ feel more positive about the services that he receives. Thank you in advance for all of your support!

- *Encourage _____ to attend speech sessions.*
- *Make speech therapy sound like a fun and enjoyable place to go: "Wow, you are so lucky; you get to see Mrs. _____ for speech."*
- *Never embarrass _____ by calling attention to his speech in front of other children.*
- *Use hand signals whenever possible to cue _____ regarding speech or provide feedback in a more private environment.*
- *With an older child, discuss speech attendance and practice as a responsibility.*
- *Attend Individualized Education Program (IEP) meetings to stay abreast of the child's progress and continued needs.*
- *Make the classroom environment a safe place to communicate.*
- *Never allow other children to tease _____ about his speech.*

If you have any questions or concerns, please contact me by phone _____ _____ or e-mail _____. You are always welcome to stop by my office/room.

_____

Speech–Language Pathologist

TEACHING SELF-MONITORING AND SELF-CORRECTING SKILLS

Self-control or self-monitoring skills have become increasingly important in promoting maintenance of clinically established skills. In the context of articulation and phonological treatment, *self-control* refers to the child's skill in *monitoring* and *correcting* his or her own sound productions without continual cueing or prompting from others. It is important to teach this skill and make it functionally independent of constant feedback. The child who self-monitors and self-corrects will have a better chance of maintaining correct articulation than the one who has not learned this skill.

The clinician can teach self-monitoring and self-correcting skills by having the child identify his own correct and incorrect productions. The clinician may ask the child to chart his or her own productions on a tally sheet and document his performance on a progress chart. We have also found it useful to audiotape or videotape portions of therapy sessions for self-control training. Some children may not be able to identify their errors until they literally "see" or "hear" them with their own eyes and ears. The child also may be trained to stop as soon as he or she notices an error.

Some children may always have to carefully monitor themselves to ensure correct production of sounds. Thus, it is imperative that the clinician considers self-monitoring and self-correcting skills as important target behaviors for training if the child does not demonstrate the spontaneous development of such skills. In our own clinical practice, we often write short-term objectives that reflect such training (e.g., "By _____, Joey will self-monitor and self-correct incorrect production of /r/ with at least 90% accuracy in conversational speech in therapy, at home, and in the classroom"). The development of such goals is particularly important with the child who is highly dependent on external support by the clinician and others for the correct production of target sounds.

The clinician can use *"My Personal Goals in Speech Therapy" Contract Form* as a "contract" between the child and those involved in helping him achieve correct production of sounds. The contract may increase the child's awareness of the goals of therapy and hopefully his self-monitoring skills. The clinician may alter the contract to meet the child's age, comprehension, and intellectual sophistication.

"My Personal Goals in Speech Therapy" Contract Form

My name is: _____

My therapy schedule is: _____

I have trouble saying the following sound(s): _____

My goal(s) for this month/semester/year is/are: _____

_____

_____

_____

I plan to reach my goal(s) by doing the following:

1. _____

2. _____

3. _____

4. _____

5. _____

_____

_____

_____

_____

The people who will help me reach my goal(s) are:

1. Me

2. Speech–Language Therapist

3. _____

4. _____

5. _____

_____

_____

Plan review date: _____

Student's signature: _____   Date: _____

Clinician's signature: _____   Date: _____

Other: _____   Date: _____

Other: _____   Date: _____

References

Bankson, J. E., & Bernthal, N. W. (1990). *Quick screen of phonology*. Chicago: Riverside Press.

Bleile, K. M. (1995). *Manual of articulation and phonological disorders: Infancy through adulthood*. San Diego, CA: Singular Publishing Group.

Edwards, H. T. (2003). *Applied phonetics: The sounds of American English* (3rd ed.). Albany, NY: Thomson Delmar Learning.

Fletcher, S. G. (1972). Time-by-count measurement of diadochokinetic syllable rate. *Journal of Speech and Hearing Research, 15*, 763–770.

Fletcher, S. G. (1978). *Time-by-count measurement of diadochokinetic syllable rate*. Austin, TX: PRO-ED.

Garbutt, C. W., & Anderson, J. O. (1980). *Effective methods for correcting articulatory defects*. Danville, IL: Interstate Printers & Publishers.

Goldman, R., & Fristoe, M. (2000). *The Goldman-Fristoe test of articulation* (2nd ed.). Circle Pines, MN: American Guidance Service.

Hodson, B. W., & Paden, E. P. (1991). *Targeting intelligible speech: A phonological approach to remediation* (2nd ed.). Austin, TX: PRO-ED.

Khan, L., & Lewis, N. (2002). *The Khan-Lewis phonological assessment* (2nd ed.). Circle Pines, MN: American Guidance Service.

McReynolds, L., & Elbert, M. (1981). Criteria for phonological process analysis. *Journal of Speech and Hearing Disorders, 46*, 197–204.

Medlin, V. L. (1975). *Handbook for speech therapy*. Austin, TX: PRO-ED.

Nemoy, E., & Davis, S. (1980). *The correction of defective consonant sounds* (16th printing). Londonderry, NH: Expression.

Peña-Brooks, A., & Hegde, M. N. (2007). *Assessment and treatment of articulation and phonological disorders in children: A dual-level text* (2nd ed.). Austin, TX: PRO-ED.

Secord, W. (1981). *T-MAC: Test of minimal articulation competence*. San Antonio, TX: Psychological Corporation.

Shriberg, L. D., & Kwiatkowski, J. (1983). Computer-assisted natural process analysis (NPA): Recent issues and data. *Seminars in Speech and Language, 4*, 397–406.

Stemple, J. C., & Holcomb, B. (1988). *Effective voice and articulation*. Columbus, OH: Merrill.

Weiss, C. E., Gordon, M. E., & Lillywhite, H. S. (1987). *Clinical management of articulatory and phonologic disorders* (2nd ed.). Baltimore, MD: Williams & Wilkins.